CMAA Exam

SECRETS

Study Guide
Your Key to Exam Success

CMAA Test Review for the Certified
Medical Administrative Assistant Exam

Dear Future Exam Success Story:

First of all, **THANK YOU** for purchasing Mometrix study materials!

Second, congratulations! You are one of the few determined test-takers who are committed to doing whatever it takes to excel on your exam. **You have come to the right place.** We developed these study materials with one goal in mind: to deliver you the information you need in a format that's concise and easy to use.

In addition to optimizing your guide for the content of the test, we've outlined our recommended steps for breaking down the preparation process into small, attainable goals so you can make sure you stay on track.

We've also analyzed the entire test-taking process, identifying the most common pitfalls and showing how you can overcome them and be ready for any curveball the test throws you.

Standardized testing is one of the biggest obstacles on your road to success, which only increases the importance of doing well in the high-pressure, high-stakes environment of test day. Your results on this test could have a significant impact on your future, and this guide provides the information and practical advice to help you achieve your full potential on test day.

Your success is our success

We would love to hear from you! If you would like to share the story of your exam success or if you have any questions or comments in regard to our products, please contact us at **800-673-8175** or **support@mometrix.com**.

Thanks again for your business and we wish you continued success!

Sincerely,
The Mometrix Test Preparation Team

Need more help? Check out our flashcards at: http://MometrixFlashcards.com/cmaa

TABLE OF CONTENTS

Introduction

Thank you for purchasing this resource! You have made the choice to prepare yourself for a test that could have a huge impact on your future, and this guide is designed to help you be fully ready for test day. Obviously, it's important to have a solid understanding of the test material, but you also need to be prepared for the unique environment and stressors of the test, so that you can perform to the best of your abilities.

For this purpose, the first section that appears in this guide is the **Secret Keys**. We've devoted countless hours to meticulously researching what works and what doesn't, and we've boiled down our findings to the five most impactful steps you can take to improve your performance on the test. We start at the beginning with study planning and move through the preparation process, all the way to the testing strategies that will help you get the most out of what you know when you're finally sitting in front of the test.

We recommend that you start preparing for your test as far in advance as possible. However, if you've bought this guide as a last-minute study resource and only have a few days before your test, we recommend that you skip over the first two Secret Keys since they address a long-term study plan.

If you struggle with **test anxiety**, we strongly encourage you to check out our recommendations for how you can overcome it. Test anxiety is a formidable foe, but it can be beaten, and we want to make sure you have the tools you need to defeat it.

Secret Key #1 – Plan Big, Study Small

There's a lot riding on your performance. If you want to ace this test, you're going to need to keep your skills sharp and the material fresh in your mind. You need a plan that lets you review everything you need to know while still fitting in your schedule. We'll break this strategy down into three categories.

Information Organization

Start with the information you already have: the official test outline. From this, you can make a complete list of all the concepts you need to cover before the test. Organize these concepts into groups that can be studied together, and create a list of any related vocabulary you need to learn so you can brush up on any difficult terms. You'll want to keep this vocabulary list handy once you actually start studying since you may need to add to it along the way.

Time Management

Once you have your set of study concepts, decide how to spread them out over the time you have left before the test. Break your study plan into small, clear goals so you have a manageable task for each day and know exactly what you're doing. Then just focus on one small step at a time. When you manage your time this way, you don't need to spend hours at a time studying. Studying a small block of content for a short period each day helps you retain information better and avoid stressing over how much you have left to do. You can relax knowing that you have a plan to cover everything in time. In order for this strategy to be effective though, you have to start studying early and stick to your schedule. Avoid the exhaustion and futility that comes from last-minute cramming!

Study Environment

The environment you study in has a big impact on your learning. Studying in a coffee shop, while probably more enjoyable, is not likely to be as fruitful as studying in a quiet room. It's important to keep distractions to a minimum. You're only planning to study for a short block of time, so make the most of it. Don't pause to check your phone or get up to find a snack. It's also important to **avoid multitasking**. Research has consistently shown that multitasking will make your studying dramatically less effective. Your study area should also be comfortable and well-lit so you don't have the distraction of straining your eyes or sitting on an uncomfortable chair.

The time of day you study is also important. You want to be rested and alert. Don't wait until just before bedtime. Study when you'll be most likely to comprehend and remember. Even better, if you know what time of day your test will be, set that time aside for study. That way your brain will be used to working on that subject at that specific time and you'll have a better chance of recalling information.

Finally, it can be helpful to team up with others who are studying for the same test. Your actual studying should be done in as isolated an environment as possible, but the work of organizing the information and setting up the study plan can be divided up. In between study sessions, you can discuss with your teammates the concepts that you're all studying and quiz each other on the details. Just be sure that your teammates are as serious about the test as you are. If you find that your study time is being replaced with social time, you might need to find a new team.

Secret Key #2 – Make Your Studying Count

You're devoting a lot of time and effort to preparing for this test, so you want to be absolutely certain it will pay off. This means doing more than just reading the content and hoping you can remember it on test day. It's important to make every minute of study count. There are two main areas you can focus on to make your studying count:

Retention

It doesn't matter how much time you study if you can't remember the material. You need to make sure you are retaining the concepts. To check your retention of the information you're learning, try recalling it at later times with minimal prompting. Try carrying around flashcards and glance at one or two from time to time or ask a friend who's also studying for the test to quiz you.

To enhance your retention, look for ways to put the information into practice so that you can apply it rather than simply recalling it. If you're using the information in practical ways, it will be much easier to remember. Similarly, it helps to solidify a concept in your mind if you're not only reading it to yourself but also explaining it to someone else. Ask a friend to let you teach them about a concept you're a little shaky on (or speak aloud to an imaginary audience if necessary). As you try to summarize, define, give examples, and answer your friend's questions, you'll understand the concepts better and they will stay with you longer. Finally, step back for a big picture view and ask yourself how each piece of information fits with the whole subject. When you link the different concepts together and see them working together as a whole, it's easier to remember the individual components.

Finally, practice showing your work on any multi-step problems, even if you're just studying. Writing out each step you take to solve a problem will help solidify the process in your mind, and you'll be more likely to remember it during the test.

Modality

Modality simply refers to the means or method by which you study. Choosing a study modality that fits your own individual learning style is crucial. No two people learn best in exactly the same way, so it's important to know your strengths and use them to your advantage.

For example, if you learn best by visualization, focus on visualizing a concept in your mind and draw an image or a diagram. Try color-coding your notes, illustrating them, or creating symbols that will trigger your mind to recall a learned concept. If you learn best by hearing or discussing information, find a study partner who learns the same way or read aloud to yourself. Think about how to put the information in your own words. Imagine that you are giving a lecture on the topic and record yourself so you can listen to it later.

For any learning style, flashcards can be helpful. Organize the information so you can take advantage of spare moments to review. Underline key words or phrases. Use different colors for different categories. Mnemonic devices (such as creating a short list in which every item starts with the same letter) can also help with retention. Find what works best for you and use it to store the information in your mind most effectively and easily.

Secret Key #3 – Practice the Right Way

Your success on test day depends not only on how many hours you put into preparing, but also on whether you prepared the right way. It's good to check along the way to see if your studying is paying off. One of the most effective ways to do this is by taking practice tests to evaluate your progress. Practice tests are useful because they show exactly where you need to improve. Every time you take a practice test, pay special attention to these three groups of questions:

- The questions you got wrong
- The questions you had to guess on, even if you guessed right
- The questions you found difficult or slow to work through

This will show you exactly what your weak areas are, and where you need to devote more study time. Ask yourself why each of these questions gave you trouble. Was it because you didn't understand the material? Was it because you didn't remember the vocabulary? Do you need more repetitions on this type of question to build speed and confidence? Dig into those questions and figure out how you can strengthen your weak areas as you go back to review the material.

Additionally, many practice tests have a section explaining the answer choices. It can be tempting to read the explanation and think that you now have a good understanding of the concept. However, an explanation likely only covers part of the question's broader context. Even if the explanation makes sense, **go back and investigate** every concept related to the question until you're positive you have a thorough understanding.

As you go along, keep in mind that the practice test is just that: practice. Memorizing these questions and answers will not be very helpful on the actual test because it is unlikely to have any of the same exact questions. If you only know the right answers to the sample questions, you won't be prepared for the real thing. **Study the concepts** until you understand them fully, and then you'll be able to answer any question that shows up on the test.

It's important to wait on the practice tests until you're ready. If you take a test on your first day of study, you may be overwhelmed by the amount of material covered and how much you need to learn. Work up to it gradually.

On test day, you'll need to be prepared for answering questions, managing your time, and using the test-taking strategies you've learned. It's a lot to balance, like a mental marathon that will have a big impact on your future. Like training for a marathon, you'll need to start slowly and work your way up. When test day arrives, you'll be ready.

Start with the strategies you've read in the first two Secret Keys—plan your course and study in the way that works best for you. If you have time, consider using multiple study resources to get different approaches to the same concepts. It can be helpful to see difficult concepts from more than one angle. Then find a good source for practice tests. Many times, the test website will suggest potential study resources or provide sample tests.

Practice Test Strategy

If you're able to find at least three practice tests, we recommend this strategy:

Untimed and Open-Book Practice

Take the first test with no time constraints and with your notes and study guide handy. Take your time and focus on applying the strategies you've learned.

Timed and Open-Book Practice

Take the second practice test open-book as well, but set a timer and practice pacing yourself to finish in time.

Timed and Closed-Book Practice

Take any other practice tests as if it were test day. Set a timer and put away your study materials. Sit at a table or desk in a quiet room, imagine yourself at the testing center, and answer questions as quickly and accurately as possible.

Keep repeating timed and closed-book tests on a regular basis until you run out of practice tests or it's time for the actual test. Your mind will be ready for the schedule and stress of test day, and you'll be able to focus on recalling the material you've learned.

Secret Key #4 – Pace Yourself

Once you're fully prepared for the material on the test, your biggest challenge on test day will be managing your time. Just knowing that the clock is ticking can make you panic even if you have plenty of time left. Work on pacing yourself so you can build confidence against the time constraints of the exam. Pacing is a difficult skill to master, especially in a high-pressure environment, so **practice is vital**.

Set time expectations for your pace based on how much time is available. For example, if a section has 60 questions and the time limit is 30 minutes, you know you have to average 30 seconds or less per question in order to answer them all. Although 30 seconds is the hard limit, set 25 seconds per question as your goal, so you reserve extra time to spend on harder questions. When you budget extra time for the harder questions, you no longer have any reason to stress when those questions take longer to answer.

Don't let this time expectation distract you from working through the test at a calm, steady pace, but keep it in mind so you don't spend too much time on any one question. Recognize that taking extra time on one question you don't understand may keep you from answering two that you do understand later in the test. If your time limit for a question is up and you're still not sure of the answer, mark it and move on, and come back to it later if the time and the test format allow. If the testing format doesn't allow you to return to earlier questions, just make an educated guess; then put it out of your mind and move on.

On the easier questions, be careful not to rush. It may seem wise to hurry through them so you have more time for the challenging ones, but it's not worth missing one if you know the concept and just didn't take the time to read the question fully. Work efficiently but make sure you understand the question and have looked at all of the answer choices, since more than one may seem right at first.

Even if you're paying attention to the time, you may find yourself a little behind at some point. You should speed up to get back on track, but do so wisely. Don't panic; just take a few seconds less on each question until you're caught up. Don't guess without thinking, but do look through the answer choices and eliminate any you know are wrong. If you can get down to two choices, it is often worthwhile to guess from those. Once you've chosen an answer, move on and don't dwell on any that you skipped or had to hurry through. If a question was taking too long, chances are it was one of the harder ones, so you weren't as likely to get it right anyway.

On the other hand, if you find yourself getting ahead of schedule, it may be beneficial to slow down a little. The more quickly you work, the more likely you are to make a careless mistake that will affect your score. You've budgeted time for each question, so don't be afraid to spend that time. Practice an efficient but careful pace to get the most out of the time you have.

Secret Key #5 – Have a Plan for Guessing

When you're taking the test, you may find yourself stuck on a question. Some of the answer choices seem better than others, but you don't see the one answer choice that is obviously correct. What do you do?

The scenario described above is very common, yet most test takers have not effectively prepared for it. Developing and practicing a plan for guessing may be one of the single most effective uses of your time as you get ready for the exam.

In developing your plan for guessing, there are three questions to address:

- When should you start the guessing process?
- How should you narrow down the choices?
- Which answer should you choose?

When to Start the Guessing Process

Unless your plan for guessing is to select C every time (which, despite its merits, is not what we recommend), you need to leave yourself enough time to apply your answer elimination strategies. Since you have a limited amount of time for each question, that means that if you're going to give yourself the best shot at guessing correctly, you have to decide quickly whether or not you will guess.

Of course, the best-case scenario is that you don't have to guess at all, so first, see if you can answer the question based on your knowledge of the subject and basic reasoning skills. Focus on the key words in the question and try to jog your memory of related topics. Give yourself a chance to bring the knowledge to mind, but once you realize that you don't have (or you can't access) the knowledge you need to answer the question, it's time to start the guessing process.

It's almost always better to start the guessing process too early than too late. It only takes a few seconds to remember something and answer the question from knowledge. Carefully eliminating wrong answer choices takes longer. Plus, going through the process of eliminating answer choices can actually help jog your memory.

Summary: Start the guessing process as soon as you decide that you can't answer the question based on your knowledge.

How to Narrow Down the Choices

The next chapter in this book (**Test-Taking Strategies**) includes a wide range of strategies for how to approach questions and how to look for answer choices to eliminate. You will definitely want to read those carefully, practice them, and figure out which ones work best for you. Here though, we're going to address a mindset rather than a particular strategy.

Your chances of guessing an answer correctly depend on how many options you are choosing from.

How many choices you have	How likely you are to guess correctly
5	20%
4	25%
3	33%
2	50%
1	100%

You can see from this chart just how valuable it is to be able to eliminate incorrect answers and make an educated guess, but there are two things that many test takers do that cause them to miss out on the benefits of guessing:

- Accidentally eliminating the correct answer
- Selecting an answer based on an impression

We'll look at the first one here, and the second one in the next section.

To avoid accidentally eliminating the correct answer, we recommend a thought exercise called **the $5 challenge**. In this challenge, you only eliminate an answer choice from contention if you are willing to bet $5 on it being wrong. Why $5? Five dollars is a small but not insignificant amount of money. It's an amount you could afford to lose but wouldn't want to throw away. And while losing $5 once might not hurt too much, doing it twenty times will set you back $100. In the same way, each small decision you make—eliminating a choice here, guessing on a question there—won't by itself impact your score very much, but when you put them all together, they can make a big difference. By holding each answer choice elimination decision to a higher standard, you can reduce the risk of accidentally eliminating the correct answer.

The $5 challenge can also be applied in a positive sense: If you are willing to bet $5 that an answer choice *is* correct, go ahead and mark it as correct.

Summary: Only eliminate an answer choice if you are willing to bet $5 that it is wrong.

Which Answer to Choose

You're taking the test. You've run into a hard question and decided you'll have to guess. You've eliminated all the answer choices you're willing to bet $5 on. Now you have to pick an answer. Why do we even need to talk about this? Why can't you just pick whichever one you feel like when the time comes?

The answer to these questions is that if you don't come into the test with a plan, you'll rely on your impression to select an answer choice, and if you do that, you risk falling into a trap. The test writers know that everyone who takes their test will be guessing on some of the questions, so they intentionally write wrong answer choices to seem plausible. You still have to pick an answer though, and if the wrong answer choices are designed to look right, how can you ever be sure that you're not falling for their trap? The best solution we've found to this dilemma is to take the decision out of your hands entirely. Here is the process we recommend:

Once you've eliminated any choices that you are confident (willing to bet $5) are wrong, select the first remaining choice as your answer.

Whether you choose to select the first remaining choice, the second, or the last, the important thing is that you use some preselected standard. Using this approach guarantees that you will not be enticed into selecting an answer choice that looks right, because you are not basing your decision on how the answer choices look.

This is not meant to make you question your knowledge. Instead, it is to help you recognize the difference between your knowledge and your impressions. There's a huge difference between thinking an answer is right because of what you know, and thinking an answer is right because it looks or sounds like it should be right.

Summary: To ensure that your selection is appropriately random, make a predetermined selection from among all answer choices you have not eliminated.

Test-Taking Strategies

This section contains a list of test-taking strategies that you may find helpful as you work through the test. By taking what you know and applying logical thought, you can maximize your chances of answering any question correctly!

It is very important to realize that every question is different and every person is different: no single strategy will work on every question, and no single strategy will work for every person. That's why we've included all of them here, so you can try them out and determine which ones work best for different types of questions and which ones work best for you.

Question Strategies

Read Carefully

Read the question and answer choices carefully. Don't miss the question because you misread the terms. You have plenty of time to read each question thoroughly and make sure you understand what is being asked. Yet a happy medium must be attained, so don't waste too much time. You must read carefully, but efficiently.

Contextual Clues

Look for contextual clues. If the question includes a word you are not familiar with, look at the immediate context for some indication of what the word might mean. Contextual clues can often give you all the information you need to decipher the meaning of an unfamiliar word. Even if you can't determine the meaning, you may be able to narrow down the possibilities enough to make a solid guess at the answer to the question.

Prefixes

If you're having trouble with a word in the question or answer choices, try dissecting it. Take advantage of every clue that the word might include. Prefixes and suffixes can be a huge help. Usually they allow you to determine a basic meaning. Pre- means before, post- means after, pro - is positive, de- is negative. From prefixes and suffixes, you can get an idea of the general meaning of the word and try to put it into context.

Hedge Words

Watch out for critical hedge words, such as *likely, may, can, sometimes, often, almost, mostly, usually, generally, rarely,* and *sometimes.* Question writers insert these hedge phrases to cover every possibility. Often an answer choice will be wrong simply because it leaves no room for exception. Be on guard for answer choices that have definitive words such as *exactly* and *always.*

Switchback Words

Stay alert for *switchbacks.* These are the words and phrases frequently used to alert you to shifts in thought. The most common switchback words are *but, although,* and *however.* Others include *nevertheless, on the other hand, even though, while, in spite of, despite, regardless of.* Switchback words are important to catch because they can change the direction of the question or an answer choice.

Face Value

When in doubt, use common sense. Accept the situation in the problem at face value. Don't read too much into it. These problems will not require you to make wild assumptions. If you have to go beyond creativity and warp time or space in order to have an answer choice fit the question, then you should move on and consider the other answer choices. These are normal problems rooted in reality. The applicable relationship or explanation may not be readily apparent, but it is there for you to figure out. Use your common sense to interpret anything that isn't clear.

Answer Choice Strategies

Answer Selection

The most thorough way to pick an answer choice is to identify and eliminate wrong answers until only one is left, then confirm it is the correct answer. Sometimes an answer choice may immediately seem right, but be careful. The test writers will usually put more than one reasonable answer choice on each question, so take a second to read all of them and make sure that the other choices are not equally obvious. As long as you have time left, it is better to read every answer choice than to pick the first one that looks right without checking the others.

Answer Choice Families

An answer choice family consists of two (in rare cases, three) answer choices that are very similar in construction and cannot all be true at the same time. If you see two answer choices that are direct opposites or parallels, one of them is usually the correct answer. For instance, if one answer choice says that quantity x increases and another either says that quantity x decreases (opposite) or says that quantity y increases (parallel), then those answer choices would fall into the same family. An answer choice that doesn't match the construction of the answer choice family is more likely to be incorrect. Most questions will not have answer choice families, but when they do appear, you should be prepared to recognize them.

Eliminate Answers

Eliminate answer choices as soon as you realize they are wrong, but make sure you consider all possibilities. If you are eliminating answer choices and realize that the last one you are left with is also wrong, don't panic. Start over and consider each choice again. There may be something you missed the first time that you will realize on the second pass.

Avoid Fact Traps

Don't be distracted by an answer choice that is factually true but doesn't answer the question. You are looking for the choice that answers the question. Stay focused on what the question is asking for so you don't accidentally pick an answer that is true but incorrect. Always go back to the question and make sure the answer choice you've selected actually answers the question and is not merely a true statement.

Extreme Statements

In general, you should avoid answers that put forth extreme actions as standard practice or proclaim controversial ideas as established fact. An answer choice that states the "process should be used in certain situations, if..." is much more likely to be correct than one that states the "process should be discontinued completely." The first is a calm rational statement and doesn't even make a

- 11 -

definitive, uncompromising stance, using a hedge word *if* to provide wiggle room, whereas the second choice is a radical idea and far more extreme.

Benchmark

As you read through the answer choices and you come across one that seems to answer the question well, mentally select that answer choice. This is not your final answer, but it's the one that will help you evaluate the other answer choices. The one that you selected is your benchmark or standard for judging each of the other answer choices. Every other answer choice must be compared to your benchmark. That choice is correct until proven otherwise by another answer choice beating it. If you find a better answer, then that one becomes your new benchmark. Once you've decided that no other choice answers the question as well as your benchmark, you have your final answer.

Predict the Answer

Before you even start looking at the answer choices, it is often best to try to predict the answer. When you come up with the answer on your own, it is easier to avoid distractions and traps because you will know exactly what to look for. The right answer choice is unlikely to be word-for-word what you came up with, but it should be a close match. Even if you are confident that you have the right answer, you should still take the time to read each option before moving on.

General Strategies

Tough Questions

If you are stumped on a problem or it appears too hard or too difficult, don't waste time. Move on! Remember though, if you can quickly check for obviously incorrect answer choices, your chances of guessing correctly are greatly improved. Before you completely give up, at least try to knock out a couple of possible answers. Eliminate what you can and then guess at the remaining answer choices before moving on.

Check Your Work

Since you will probably not know every term listed and the answer to every question, it is important that you get credit for the ones that you do know. Don't miss any questions through careless mistakes. If at all possible, try to take a second to look back over your answer selection and make sure you've selected the correct answer choice and haven't made a costly careless mistake (such as marking an answer choice that you didn't mean to mark). This quick double check should more than pay for itself in caught mistakes for the time it costs.

Pace Yourself

It's easy to be overwhelmed when you're looking at a page full of questions; your mind is confused and full of random thoughts, and the clock is ticking down faster than you would like. Calm down and maintain the pace that you have set for yourself. Especially as you get down to the last few minutes of the test, don't let the small numbers on the clock make you panic. As long as you are on track by monitoring your pace, you are guaranteed to have time for each question.

Don't Rush

It is very easy to make errors when you are in a hurry. Maintaining a fast pace in answering questions is pointless if it makes you miss questions that you would have gotten right otherwise. Test writers like to include distracting information and wrong answers that seem right. Taking a little extra time to avoid careless mistakes can make all the difference in your test score. Find a pace that allows you to be confident in the answers that you select.

Keep Moving

Panicking will not help you pass the test, so do your best to stay calm and keep moving. Taking deep breaths and going through the answer elimination steps you practiced can help to break through a stress barrier and keep your pace.

Final Notes

The combination of a solid foundation of content knowledge and the confidence that comes from practicing your plan for applying that knowledge is the key to maximizing your performance on test day. As your foundation of content knowledge is built up and strengthened, you'll find that the strategies included in this chapter become more and more effective in helping you quickly sift through the distractions and traps of the test to isolate the correct answer.

Now it's time to move on to the test content chapters of this book, but be sure to keep your goal in mind. As you read, think about how you will be able to apply this information on the test. If you've already seen sample questions for the test and you have an idea of the question format and style, try to come up with questions of your own that you can answer based on what you're reading. This will give you valuable practice applying your knowledge in the same ways you can expect to on test day.

Good luck and good studying!

Scheduling

Appointment Scheduling

Appointments are often made by telephone although return visits may be scheduled in person while the patient is in the office. Return visits are easier to schedule because the information about the patient's insurance is already on file, and the healthcare provider has often indicated when the return visit is needed. If no appointments are available near the time the healthcare provider has indicated, then the CMAA should check with the healthcare provider to determine if a later date is acceptable. For telephone appointments, it's important to be courteous and to avoid sounding rushed or impatient. Information generally required for an appointment includes:

- Patient's name and birthdate.
- Patient's status: New or returning patient.
- Contact information: Telephone (home and/or cell), text message.
- Purpose of the visit: Needed to estimate time needed for the appointment.
- Referral or self-selected.
- Insurance coverage: Especially important for Medicaid and Medicare patients as not all healthcare providers accept assignment of benefits for Medicare or Medicaid patients.

Documents Used to Establish Identity

Documents That Can Establish Identity (Must Not Be Outdated)	
Passports	Contain photograph and further identifying information, such as name, gender, color of eyes and hair, and weight.
Driver's licenses	Must contain a photograph and further identifying information.
Federal, state or local government ID cards	Must contain a photograph and further identifying information.
School/University ID cards	Must contain a photograph and person's name.
Voter registration card	Vary widely from one state/territory to another but should contain name and address. Some states include a photograph.
Military ID cards, including those of dependents	Contain photograph, name, pay grade/rank, affiliation, expiration date and Department of Defense ID number on the front and the date of birth, benefits number, blood type, Geneva convention category, and date of issue on the back.
Native American tribal documents	Generally, include a photograph and further information similar to a driver's license.

Types of Patient Visits

Patient visits may include:

- <u>Routine</u>: Patient presents with new or existing problems and/or health conditions, such as hypertension or diabetes.
- <u>Procedure-associated</u>: Patient is scheduled for a procedure during the visit, such as an ultrasound or echocardiogram.
- <u>Physical exam</u>: For a complete PE, all systems are reviewed, and some diagnostic procedures, such as a CBC and ECG, may be routinely included.

- 15 -

- Non-urgent follow-up: Patient was seen previously and is following up so healthcare provider can evaluate progress/problems such as after a patient has started a new medication or to evaluate healing after surgery.
- Urgent/acute illness: Patient has acute problems and may need immediate care.
- New non-urgent problem/illness: Patient has a condition that requires assessment, diagnosis, and/or treatment.
- Sports physical: PE may require that a specific form provided by the school or organization be completed.
- Medicare Preventive Physical Exam (initial): Available to new enrollees within the first 12 months of coverage and may include preventive screening, such as for cancer, and immunizations.
- Screening/Diagnostic tests and imaging: Patient visits for specific tests or imaging.

Appointment Matrix

An **appointment matrix** is the form that the appointment schedule takes on paper or in the computer. Typically, the matrix lists the physicians and nurse practitioners or physician's assistants, the times of day (usually in 10 minute-increments and the days of the week). The appointment matrix may be quite simple (as below) or complex. Any time that a physician or nurse practitioner is not available is blocked out so that no appointments will be made at those times. If the physician or nurse practitioner sets aside certain days or times for extended visits, such as for admission history and physical, these times may be color-coded or otherwise noted. Example:

Dr. Smith	Hr.	May 15	May 16
	8:00	Mrs. Jones—BP check	Staff meeting
	8:10	Mr. Brown--Glucose	" "
	8:20	Miss White--UTI	" "
	8:30	" "	Mr. Smythe—Ulcer exam
	8:40	Telephone calls	" "

Daily Appointment Schedule

While the appointment matrix is often completed in the computer or on paper in pencil to allow for easy corrections, a **daily appointment schedule** is a legal document that must be retained for at least 5 years (and most practices store them indefinitely). The daily appointment schedule is a list of patients that are to be seen that day. It can be completed on the computer and printed or done on paper in permanent ink. Additionally, any additions or corrections to the schedule must be made in ink. No shows and cancellations should be indicated by crossing out the patient's name in red ink and making a notation as to the reason (for example, "NS" or "C"). The appointment schedule is used to pull medical records if the practice utilizes paper records or to access electronic records.

Jones Medical Practice
Daily appointment schedule for 2-8-1ⁱ

Time	Name	Telephone #	Purpose	Notes
8:00	Telephone calls			
8:15	Review lab reports			
8:30	Simms, Sarah	866-4302	Recheck—BP	10 minutes late
8:45	Jackson, James	722-6685	PE—1 yr.	Fx'd rt. Hip 8-18
9:00	" " " "	" " "		

Telephone Emergency/Urgent Requests

If a patient calls for an appointment and indicates an **emergency or urgent situation** (severe pain, bleeding, loss of consciousness, paralysis, injury, breathing difficulties, chest pain), the CMAA should try to obtain the caller's name and telephone number (in case the call is disconnected), a description of symptoms and history (onset, duration, severity), the patient's name (if different from caller), and any treatment attempted. If the problem is urgent, the CMAA should not attempt to assess the need for an appointment but should transfer the call to a triage nurse or directly to a physician so that that person can better assess need and set an appointment or refer the patient to 9-1-1. In rare instances, such as if a patient loses consciousness while calling or is too ill to call 9-1-1, the CMAA may need to call 9-1-1 on a separate line but should stay on the line and connected to the patient until emergency medical responders arrive.

Fixed Scheduling

With **fixed scheduled appointments**, each patient is generally scheduled to see the health provider at a specific time, such as at 9 AM, and no other patient is scheduled at the same time. Appointments may range from 10 minutes (or less in some practices) to 1.5 hours, depending on the patient's needs and the type of appointment. For example, a routine follow-up may be scheduled for 15 minutes, a new patient for 30 minutes, but a consultation and/or complete physical exam for 45 minutes to 1.5 hours. If patients are scheduled back-to-back with no time allowed for drop-ins, telephone consultations, emergencies, or appointments that exceed the scheduled time, a backlog of patients may begin to occur, so some extra unscheduled time should be planned into the daily schedule so that the wait time for patients is minimized and the healthcare provider does not feel pressured or rushed.

Wave Booking, Modified Wave Booking, and Tidal Wave Booking

Wave booking is scheduling 3 or 4 patients every half hour or hour so that they are all scheduled to arrive at the same time and are seen in the order in which they arrive. With this type of scheduling, extra patients can usually be easily fitted into the schedule. Wave booking assumes that some patients will require less time than others, but problems may arise if patients object to having to wait while others are seen, and wait time may increase for the last patients seen during the time slot.

Modified wave booking may take various forms, such as scheduling waves of patients on the hour and leaving the second half of the hour unscheduled to allow for drop ins and extended visits or using fixed scheduling on the hour and wave scheduling on the half hour.

Tidal wave/Open hour booking is an open time period in which anyone can come without a prescheduled appointment and is seen on a first-come, first-served basis or according to acuity, used most commonly in urgent care.

Clustering

Clustering is scheduling one type of patient or those having similar procedures only during a block of time. For example, one morning a week may be scheduled for doing breast exams. A gastroenterologist may carry out colonoscopies only two days per week. Examples of conditions/treatment that may be scheduled in clusters may include:

- Immunizations.
- Well-baby examinations.

- Routine obstetric examinations.
- Chemotherapy administration.
- Sports physicals.

With clustering, patients may have fixed scheduled appointments during the block of time or some form of wave booking may be used, depending on the type of cluster. For example, if patients are coming for immunizations, then wave booking may be used because of the short time needed, while patients for obstetric examinations may have fixed scheduling. Clustering can save time in setting up rooms and carrying out procedures because rooms and equipment needed can be easily set up in advance.

Double Booking

Double booking is scheduling two patients for the time same time period. Because double booking can result in a backlog, it is usually used only if there is a difference in acuity or needs between two patients. For example, one patient may have a minor rash and another hypertension and diabetes, so the first patient may require only a brief visit, allowing the rest of the scheduled time for the other patient. However, if extra time is needed for one or both patients, then some free time should be scheduled after the booking to allow for extended visits. Double booking is often done to fit in an emergency patient or to carry out diagnostic tests, such as an electrocardiogram, and is most often used for short visits or in practices with a high no-show rate. Double booking also may be done before noon breaks or at the end of the day so that the health provider can leave early if possible.

Scheduling Issues

No Shows and Cancellations

Patients who schedule an appointment and fail to keep the appointment without notice are classified as **no shows**, and this must be recorded on the daily appointment schedule as well as in the patient's medical record for legal reasons in the event that the patient's failure to keep the appointment results in physical or mental harm of some type. **Cancellations** on the day of the appointment should also be noted on the daily appointment schedule and medical record and the reason for the cancellation noted if known and any rescheduling information. Practices may charge a fee for no shows and cancellations under specified hours prior to an appointment, but the patient must be advised of this policy when making the appointment because a fee cannot be imposed without prior notice. Medicare and many insurers don't pay for these charges. After a specific number of no shows (such as 3 consecutive), some practices terminate the relationship with the patient, following an established protocol, such as by a certified letter with a return receipt.

Healthcare Provider Absence

In some cases, patients must be rescheduled because a **healthcare provider is ill, out of town, or unavailable** for other reasons (such as for a death in the family). Patients should be notified as soon as possible and rescheduled or given recommendations for alternative physicians or medical services (such as an emergency department) where they can receive care. Patients should be advised only that the healthcare provider will be out of the office and unavailable. Reporting that the healthcare provider is ill is a HIPAA violation unless the healthcare provider has explicitly instructed staff to notify patients of the illness, but this is usually only the case with extended illnesses. Patients should not be advised if the healthcare provider is out of town as this may increase the risk of break-ins to the healthcare provider's home for practice. In a practice where the healthcare providers must be on call during office hours, such as obstetricians, the patient may be told the reason: "The doctor is delivering a baby."

Extended Wait Time

Extended wait time is common in medical practice and a common cause of complaints from patients. The CMAA should always address the issue directly if patients have to wait because patients may become increasingly annoyed or stressed if the situation is ignored. Steps include:

- Acknowledging the extended wait, providing an explanation, and apologizing for the inconvenience.
- Estimating the additional wait time.
- Giving patients options (if possible), such as returning at a later time or rescheduling.
- Offering comfort measures, such as water, reading material, or (for children) toys or other activities.

Even if the patient or family responds negatively to interventions, it's important to remain supportive and professional and to refrain from responding negatively in return. If extended wait time is a common occurrence in a practice, then the scheduling practices should be reexamined to determine the cause and modifications made in scheduling if possible.

Walk-in Patients

Occasionally patients **walk in** to make an appointment. If there is no free time in the schedule and the situation is not urgent, then it's appropriate to explain that there are no openings and to offer to make an appointment for a later time. If the physician agrees to see a non-urgent patient, the patient should be advised to call ahead for any subsequent visits as time is not always available in the schedule to fit in extra patients. If the situation is urgent, such as a patient complaining of chest pain or shortness of breath, then the CMAA should immediately notify a nurse or physician and ask that person to assess the patient. If no nurse or physician is available, then the CMAA should say, "I will call 9-1-1" and make the patient as comfortable as possible and should stay with the patient until emergency responders arrive.

Variables

A number of **variables** must be considered when scheduling a patient for an appointment, including:

- New or returning patient: New patients may need to fill out history forms and sign a number of different documents (privacy policy, insurance forms, release forms). In some cases, the patient may be able to download the forms online or may receive forms by mail before the appointment if time allows. Returning patients may need to upgrade insurance or other information. New patients are usually scheduled for longer appointments than return visits.
- Urgency: Patients with acute problems may need immediate scheduling while others may be able to wait until a time slot is available.
- Insurance coverage: The practice may not accept the patient's insurance, or (if no insurance) the patient may have to demonstrate ability to pay, according to practice policies.
- Policies: Patients must be advised of policies regarding check-in, rescheduling, and cancellations, such as a charge if an appointment is not cancelled by a certain time period.
- Staff preferences: Staff may prefer or need scheduling at specific times.

Referrals

Because **referrals** are an important source of new patients, patients that are referred are often given priority in scheduling, according to practice policy and depending on the urgency of the referral. If the referral is made directly, as per telephone, then the CMAA should ask about urgency and obtain as much information as possible, including a request for medical records to save time later. In some cases, the patient calls after being advised to do so by a referring healthcare provider. In that case, medical records should generally be obtained in order to assess urgency before making the appointment. Three types of referrals are most common:

- Consultation: Usually to a specialist for diagnostic testing, surgery, or additional treatment. Some types of testing and treatment may require preauthorization for insurance companies.
- Therapy/Treatments: May include psychological therapy, physical therapy, occupational therapy, speech therapy. Therapy may require preauthorization for insurance companies.
- Community resources: May include home health agencies, meals programs, respite care.

Follow-up Appointments

To schedule a **follow-up appointment**, the CMAA needs to know the patient's name, contact information (email, telephone, or text), the purpose of the follow-up, and any scheduling issues that may apply. For example, dressing changes may be scheduled for 2 mornings during the week, and the physician may block out certain times from the schedule. Additionally, patients may need to be scheduled early in the morning if they are scheduled for treatment or testing that requires fasting. The CMAA should check to see what if any directions regarding the follow-up appointment are needed. For example, if the patient is to return for a colonoscopy, the patient would need the prep (or a prescription for the prep) and instructions for administration. On the appointment card, the CMAA should note the date and time and make a notation of any important factors, such as the need for fasting.

Diagnostic Procedures

To **schedule diagnostic procedures**, the CMAA should gather information about the patient and insurance and determine the diagnostic test to be scheduled and the appropriate time frame. Steps include:

1. Selecting a diagnostic center/laboratory and verifying that services are covered under the patient's insurance plan.
2. Obtaining the appropriate preauthorization is necessary or checking with the insurance company if unsure of the need for preauthorization.
3. Discussing availability and time/date preferences with patient.
4. Telephone diagnostic center/laboratory to schedule appointment.
5. Provide information to the patient regarding the place, date, and time of the diagnostic procedure.
6. Provide any pre- or post-test instructions (such as dietary restrictions, special prep) to the patient and review with the patient to make sure the patient understands.
7. Record the scheduled procedure in the patient's medical record.
8. Record the scheduled procedure in the diagnostic procedure tracking log.

In-Patient Hospitalization

When scheduling in-**patient hospitalization** for a patient, the CMAA should first gather all necessary information before calling the admitting department and should obtain preauthorization from insurance companies as needed. If a non-emergency admission, the CMAA should determine both the patient's and the physician's availability prior to scheduling. Information that the admitting department needs includes the patient's name, address, date of birth, admitting diagnosis, insurance information (primary and secondary), preauthorization number (if appropriate), and purpose of hospitalization. The CMAA should also inform the admitting department when the admitting physician plans to see the patient as the patient must be seen by his/her physician within 24 hours. In some cases, care of the patient is assumed by a hospitalist upon admission and not by the patient's personal physician. The patient must be informed of any prehospitalization testing or restrictions or other special instructions.

<u>Surgical Procedures</u>

When scheduling **surgical procedures**, which may be done as an inpatient or in an outpatient surgery center, the CMAA should first gather all necessary information: the location where the surgery is to be performed, the patient's name, the telephone number, the date of birth, the type of surgery that is to be scheduled, the timeframe, and the name of the surgeon and any assistants as well as the anesthesiologist. Additionally, the CMAA should contact the insurance company for preauthorization and obtain the preauthorization number that the surgical center will need. If preauthorization testing (PAT), such as CBC, chem-panel, chest x-ray, or ECG, is required, the CMAA must know who is to perform the testing and may need to schedule the tests as well. Patients must be provided pre-surgical instructions, such as the need to be NPO before surgery and whether or not to take medications the day of surgery or in the days prior to surgery.

<u>Consultations/Referrals</u>

When **scheduling consultations/referrals** to other healthcare providers, such as a specialist (ophthalmologist, neurologist, orthopedist), therapist (physical therapist, occupational therapist, speech therapist, recreational therapist, psychologist), or community resource (home health agency, meals-on-wheels) the CMAA should first gather all necessary information and complete the referral form. Necessary information includes the patient's name, telephone number, date of birth, admission diagnosis, and insurance information as well as the name of the referring healthcare provider and the reason for the consultation/referral. The referral includes the number of anticipated visits (such as PT three times a week for a month). Preauthorization may be required for consultations/referrals. One copy of the referral form is stored in the patient's medical record and another given to the patient or sent directly to the consultant/therapist/community resource. The patient may be instructed to make an appointment independently or the CMAA may make the initial appointment after discussing time eligibility with the patient.

<u>Sales Representatives and Other Healthcare Providers</u>

Visitors may disrupt schedules when they ask to see the healthcare provider:

- <u>Other healthcare providers</u> may drop by to confer or discuss an issue. They should be asked to wait in the office or other private room and the healthcare provider to whom they want to speak notified as soon as possible.
- <u>Sales and pharmaceutical representatives</u> often bring samples and information about new drugs, but the ACMM may need to screen them to determine if they are promoting drugs or products of interest to the practice. If so, then they should be advised of a good time to return or fitted into the schedule when time is available. If the products or drugs are not of interest to the practice, the representatives should be so advised. The healthcare provider may develop a list of representatives that the healthcare provider wants to see to save time.

<u>Decreasing No-Show Rates</u>

A medical practice can take a number of steps to **decrease no-show rates**, including asking the preferred method of contact:

- <u>Appointment cards</u>: Every patient should receive an appointment card with the date and time of the appointment whenever possible, and the card should indicate that appointments must be cancelled at least 24 hours in advance. For telephone appointments, a letter may be sent confirming the date and time of the appointment if time permits.
- <u>Telephone reminders</u>: These may be done by a staff person or may be automated. Reminders are usually sent 1 to 3 days prior to the appointment time. Automated calls may allow a response to indicate that the person plans to keep or cancel the appointment.
- <u>Emails/Text messages</u>: Some people prefer to be reminded of appointments by email or text messages.

Development of Policies

Policies must be based on best practices and conform to state, federal, and accreditation regulations and guidelines. Empowerment includes encouraging participation of all staff in policy making. Objectives for policies should be clearly outlined. In some cases, policies may be broad and cover all aspects of an organization, but in other cases, policies may be much more specific, such as a policy regarding no-shows or missed appointments. Conflict of interest policies should be in place to ensure that those involved in review activities should not be primary care givers or have an economic or personal interest in a case under review. Policies should ensure that access to protected health information be limited to those who need the information to complete duties related to direct care or performance improvement review activities. Policy and procedure manuals should be readily available organization-wide in easily accessible format, such as online. Policy issues may include cost-effectiveness, insurance coverage, criteria for qualified staff, and legal implications.

Fee Schedules

A **fee schedule** is the list of a healthcare provider's charges for services and involves consideration of expertise, time utilized, and services provided. With fee-for-service, the fee schedule is fairly straight-forward with a specific fee listed for each service, such as a fee of $30 for an annual flu shot and $100 for a comprehensive exam for a new patient. Fee schedules often correspond to the items on the encounter form. The fee schedule includes the appropriate CPT code for each item because this code is needed for billing purposes. However, many factors can affect fee schedules, and a health provider may actually have multiple fee schedules; for example, a healthcare provider may have one fee schedule for fee-for-service, another for Medicare, another for Medicaid, and

- 22 -

additional fee schedules for specific insurance companies or HMOs, based on contractual agreements. It's imperative that the right fee schedule be considered when claims are submitted.

```
Jones Medical Practice
Fee Schedule

Office visits, New patients:
   •  99201   Minimal exam:   $50.00
   •  99202   Focused exam:   $75.00
   •  99203   Comp. exam:    $100.00

Office procedures:
   •  09000   EKG, 12 lead:   $100.00
   •  90724   Influenza inj:   $30.00
```

Preauthorization for Services

Insurance carriers may require **preauthorization** for diagnostic procedures, hospitalization, and surgical procedures, and managed care programs often also require preauthorization for referrals, so determining the need for preauthorization should be part of verification of insurance benefits. Insurance cards often list a telephone number, fax number, or other contact information for preauthorization. The CMAA should gather necessary information before contacting the insurance company and fill out the preauthorization/referral form with the information:

- Patient's name and demographic information.
- Healthcare provider's name, provider identification number, address, and telephone number.
- Name of the insurance plan, address, and contact information (telephone, fax, secure email)
- Patient's preliminary diagnosis, including diagnostic codes.
- Planned procedure/referral, including procedure codes.
- Name, address and telephone number or other contact information for referrals.
- Amount of patient's copayment and/or deductible.
- Hospital benefits (inpatient and outpatient).
- Healthcare providers within the network (if applicable).

The preauthorization/referral form is usually faxed to the insurance company although in emergency situations preauthorization may be obtained by telephone.

Pre-Testing Instructions

Prior to tests or procedures that require **pre-testing instructions**, the patient should be advised regarding these instructions verbally in person or by phone to ensure that the patient receives the information and can ask questions. The patient should also be a given a copy of the printed instructions. If the patient is not present at the time, the instructions may be sent either by an email attachment or by regular mail. Any instructions regarding holding of medications or the need for a specific prep (such as for a colonoscopy) or withholding of food and drink should be emphasized. Printed instructions should be written in a simple format, such as by including bulleted lists, and in at least a 12 to 14 font for ease of reading. If pre-testing instructions include the need for specific prep, a prescription and/or a list of OTC items (such as laxatives) should be provided the patient. When and how and what type of instructions are provided patient must be documented in the medical record.

- 23 -

Diagnostic Procedure Tracking Log

The **diagnostic procedure tracking log** is used to record all diagnostic procedures that are scheduled to ensure that no results are overlooked and that patients are informed of the results of all tests. Formats may vary somewhat. For example, some forms may include procedure codes. The diagnostic procedure tracking log should be filled out immediately when procedures are scheduled and again when results are received. The log should be checked every work day at the beginning of the day and again at the end so that calls to patients are made in a timely manner and recorded.

Jones Medical Practice
Diagnostic Procedure Log

Test Date	Patient	Test	Place	Date result received	Patient informed
1-4-19	Barnes, T.C.	Colonoscopy	Colons et al	1-7-19	1-7-19
1-7-19	Mehdi, M.A.	CBC	CASC Lab	1-8-19	1-9-19
1-8-19	Giotti, A.S.	Mammogram	Mmgrphy Ctr.		

Informing Patients of Diagnostic Procedure Results

Patients should be informed of **diagnostic procedure results** as soon as possible, as patients are often anxious when awaiting results. Once test results are received and the date entered into the diagnostic procedure tracking log, the test should be reviewed by the ordering healthcare provider before the patient is notified of the results. The healthcare provider should indicate who should notify the patient. When test results are negative, the CMAA may be tasked with notifying the patient either by letter (standard format is generally utilized) or telephone. If test results are positive and/or follow-up is needed, then the ordering healthcare provider or a nurse usually contacts the patient. In some cases, the CMAA may need to make a follow-up appointment for the healthcare provider to discuss test results with the patient. For serious results, such as a positive finding of cancer, the physician should speak directly to the patient, in person if possible.

Time Management Approaches

Approaches that the CMAA can utilize for **time management** include:

- Planning ahead: Maintaining a master schedule that lists visits and meetings.
- Keeping diary/schedule up-to-date on a daily basis.
- Utilizing color coding: Using colored stickers to indicate different needs, such as red stickers for those things that require urgent attention.
- Scheduling a time to return calls: Making calls first thing in the day so that any alterations needed in the schedule can be made promptly.
- Utilizing time management and/or case management software.
- Making appropriate referrals.
- Preparing reports in advance, avoiding last minute rush.
- Making to-do lists or action plans.
- Creating templates for frequently used forms/letters.
- Filing immediately and throwing out unnecessary paperwork.
- Utilizing GPS and mapping software to plan routes when having to travel.
- Prioritizing work.
- Avoiding all procrastination.

Medical Records

<u>Documentation Purposes</u>

Documentation is a form of communication that provides information about the healthcare patient and confirms that care was provided. Accurate, objective, and complete documentation of patient care is required by both accreditation and reimbursement agencies, including federal and state governments. Purposes of documentation include:

- Carrying out professional responsibility.
- Establishing accountability.
- Communicating among health professionals.
- Educating staff.
- Providing information for research.
- Satisfying legal and practice standards.
- Ensuring reimbursement.

While documentation focuses on progress notes, there are many other aspects to charting. Doctor's orders must be noted, medication administration must be documented on medication sheets, and vital signs must be graphed. Flow sheets must be checked off, filled out, or initialed. Admission assessments may involve primarily checklists or may require extensive documentation. The primary issue in malpractice cases is inaccurate or incomplete documentation. It's better to over-document than under, but effective documentation does neither.

<u>Documentation Requirements</u>

Documentation requirements for medical records include:

- <u>Accuracy</u>: Documentation should always include any change in patient's condition, treatments, medications, or other interventions, patient responses, and any complaints of family or patient. Subjective descriptions (especially negative terms, which could be used to establish bias in court), such as tired, angry, confused, bored, rude, happy, and euphoric must be avoided and objective descriptions used.
- <u>Timeliness</u>: All treatments and interventions should be documented promptly, including the time given, but never in advance as this is illegal. Military time is used in many healthcare institutions but if standard time is used, the person documenting should always include "AM" or "PM" with time notations.
- <u>Legibility</u>: If hand entries are used, then writing should be done with a blue or black permanent ink pen and should be neat and legible, in block printing if handwriting is illegible. No pen or pencil that can be erased can be used to document in a patient's record because this could facilitate falsification of records. For the same reason, a line must be drawn through empty spaces in the documentation.
- <u>Clarity</u>: A standardized vocabulary should be used, including approved abbreviations and symbols.

<u>Methods of Documentation</u>

Different **methods of documentation** used for patients' medical records include:

- <u>Narrative</u>: This charting provides a chronological report of the patient's condition, treatment, and responses. It is an easy method of charting but may be disorganized and repetitive, and if different people are making notes, they may address different issues, making it difficult to get an overall picture of the patient's progress.

- SOAP (subjective data, objective data, assessment, plan of action): This problem-oriented form of charting includes establishing goals, expected outcomes, and needs and then compiling a numbered list of problems. A SOAP note is made for each separate problem.
  - Subjective: Patient's statement of problem.
  - Objective: Direct observation.
  - Assessment: Determination of possible causes.
  - Plan: Short- and long-range goals and immediate plan of care.
- PIE (problem, intervention, evaluation): This problem-oriented form of charting is similar to SOAP but less complex. It combines use of flow sheets with progress notes and a list of problems. Each problem is numbered sequentially and a PIE note is made for each problem, at least one time daily (or during treatment, depending on the frequency).
- Focus/DAR (data, action, response): This type of focused charting includes documentation about health problems, changes in condition, and concerns or events, focusing on data about the injury/illness, the action taken by the healthcare provider, and the response. The written format is usually in 3 columns (D-A-R) rather than traditional narrative linear form. A DAR note is used for each focus item.

If there are multiple problems (edema, pain, restricted activity, etc.,), this charting can be very time-consuming, as each element of SOAP must be addressed. SOAP notes may be extended to SOAPIER (including intervention, evaluation, and revision.)

The **CHEDDAR** method of documentation is used by many medical practices for problem-oriented medical records:

C	Chief complaint	Patient's subjective description and presenting problems.
H	History	Onset of problem and duration and contributing factors (social, physical, psychological)
E	Examination	Objective findings based on physical assessment.
D	Details of problem/complaint	Details regarding the chief complaint.
D	Drugs and dosages	List of all current prescribed medications, OTC medications, and supplements as well as dosages.
A	Assessment	Final assessment based on observations.
R	Return visit information (if applies)	Need for return visit or further treatment.

Following up to Ensure Patient Compliance

Because patients are often non-compliant with physician's instructions because of misunderstanding, lack of motivation, or lack of sufficient funds, it's important to **follow-up** to ensure compliance. Steps include:

1. Reviewing instructions with patient and encouraging questions.
2. Asking the patient's preferred method of contact (telephone, email, text message) and making a notation on the medical record.
3. Advising the patient that a follow-up contact will be made to see how the patient is progressing.
4. Logging the name and contact information and date of needed follow-up in the appropriate log or record to ensure follow-up is done in a timely manner.

5. Contacting the patient to determine if the patient is following instructions and has any questions. If not, explaining the rationale for doing so. If so, providing positive feedback.
6. Informing the healthcare provider of any problems.
7. Documenting the contact and patient's response in the medical record.

HIPAA

The **Health Insurance Portability and Accountability Act** (HIPAA) addresses the rights of the individual related to privacy of health information. Healthcare providers must not release any information or documentation about a patient's condition or treatment without consent, as the individual has the right to determine who has access to personal information. Personal information about the patient is considered protected health information (PHI), and consists of any identifying or personal information about the patient, such as health history, condition, or treatments in any form, and any documentation, including electronic, verbal, or written. Personal information can be shared with spouse, legal guardians, parents, those with durable power of attorney for the patient, and those involved in care of the patient, such as physicians, without a specific release, but the patient should always be consulted if personal information is to be discussed with others present to ensure there is no objection. Failure to comply with HIPAA regulations can make a healthcare provider liable for legal and civil action. Patients should be provided written privacy policies on admission so that they are aware of their rights.

Verification of Insurance Benefits

Verification of insurance benefits should be carried out before the patient is seen by the healthcare provider. In some cases, an up-to-date insurance card may be sufficient, but in many cases, such as Medicaid and managed care programs, benefits must be verified. Each practice should establish protocols, but in general the steps include:

1. Ask for the insurance card and make photocopies, front and back, noting the need for copayment: "You have a copayment of $20. How would you like to pay that?"
2. Run the card through a point-of-service insurance verification device, if available, OR
3. Contact the insurance company directly by telephone to determine eligibility, exclusions, and types of preauthorization needed.
4. Record the name, title, and contact number for the insurance representative who provided information in case problems arise.
5. Record information regarding verification on a benefits verification form and in the patient's medical record.
6. Ask patient to sign a Patient Responsibility Notification form that outlines common requirements and patient's responsibilities regarding insurance benefits.

Patient Intake

Verifying Identification and Confirming Demographic Information

When **verifying identification**, the first thing to do is to ask the patient's name, including the first name, middle name or initial, and the last name as well as the patient's birthdate as more than one patient may have the same name. A passport or driver's license with a photo should be checked to verify that the person is who he/she claims to be, keeping in mind that people's appearance may change somewhat over time and that weight and hair color may be different. Some practices now routinely ask permission to take patients' pictures and include them in the medical record as a further method of verifying identification. Patients should be asked to fill out a registration form that includes **demographic information** including insurance information at the first visit, but should be asked at every subsequent visit if any information has changed, and any changes noted in the patient's medical record.

Advance Directives

In accordance to Federal and state laws, individuals have the right to self-determination in health care, including decisions about end of life care through **advance directives** such as living wills and the right to assign a surrogate person to make decisions through a **durable power of attorney**. Patients should routinely be questioned about an advanced directive as they may present at a healthcare organization without the document. Patients who have indicated they desire a **do-not-resuscitate** (DNR) order should not receive resuscitative treatments for terminal illness or conditions in which meaningful recovery cannot occur. Patients and families of those with terminal illnesses should be questioned as to whether the patients are Hospice patients. For those with DNR requests or those withdrawing life support, healthcare providers should provide the patient palliative rather than curative measures, such as pain control and/or oxygen, and emotional support to the patient and family. Religious traditions and beliefs about death should be treated with respect.

PHI

Sensitive information is classified under HIPAA as **protected health information** (PHI) and includes

- Any information about an individual's past, present, or future health or condition (mental or physical).
- Provision of health care provided to the individual
- Any information related to payment for healthcare services that can be used to identify the person.
- Identifying information: Name, address, Social Security number, birthdate) and any document or material that contains the identifying information (such as laboratory records).

Information that is to be shared or aggregated for research purposes must first be de-identified. The HIPAA privacy rule provides two methods of de-identification:

- Expert determination (based on applying statistical or scientific principles): The expert must have appropriate knowledge and must document the method and analysis results.
- Safe harbor (removing 18 types of identifiers): Includes names, geographic information, zip codes, telephone numbers, license numbers, account numbers, Fax numbers, serial numbers of devices, email addresses, URLs, full-face photographs, - year) and biometric identifiers.

Patients with Special Needs

Hearing Impaired

Hearing impaired patients may have some hearing and may use hearing aids while deaf patients typically have little or no hearing. Some patients are able to use lip reading to various degrees, so the CMAA should always face the patient (at 3-6 feet) and speak slowly and clearly, using gestures (not excessively) to augment speech:

- Hearing impaired: Assistive devices (hearing aids, writing material) should be available and used during communication. Use a normal tone of voice and speak in short sentences. Minimize environmental noises.
- Deaf: If patients are deaf, sign language interpreters should be used for important communication (face the patient, not the interpreter). Assistive devices, such as writing materials, TDD phone/relay service, should be available for use. Always announce presence on entering a room by waving, clapping, tapping the foot (whatever works best for the patient). Ensure alarms have visual feedback (lights). Do not chew, smoke, or eat while speaking to the patient.

Visually Impaired

Visual impairment is unrelated to intelligence or hearing, so the CMAA should speak with age-appropriate vocabulary in a normal tone of voice, facing the patient so the CMAA can observe facial expression. Depending on the degree of visual impairment, the patient may not be able to see gestures or materials; so alternate forms of materials (braille handouts or enlarged text) or manipulatives must be considered. The field of vision may be impaired so that the patient sees shapes or has better vision in some areas than others, and the CMAA should try to position herself/himself for the patient's advantage. The CMAA should also announce his/her presence, explain actions and movement ("I'm putting your dressing supplies on the counter."), announce position ("I'm at your right side.") and always tell the patient if intending to touch the patient ("I'm going to take your blood pressure on your right arm").

Intellectually Disabled and Illiterate

Communicating with patients who are **intellectually disabled** can be challenging, and patients may have very different and individual responses, so observation of the patient must serve as a guide. Patients may be apprehensive and frightened, so the CMAA should maintain a friendly normal tone of voice and should speak with the patient often to establish rapport, even if the response is not clear. The CMAA should always ask the patient before touching his/her things. Initiating communication by talking about familiar things (family, pictures, the past) may be comforting for the patient. If responses are unclear or inappropriate, the CMAA can say, "I didn't understand that" but should not laugh or indicate frustration. A guardian may be responsible for authorizing care. Communicating with patients who are **illiterate** is not different than with most patients because the patients may be quite intelligent, but the CMAA should take care to explain procedures and provide verbal and pictorial information rather than written instructions.

Language Barriers

Language barriers, such as when a patient does not speak English, may interfere with communication. If a patient does not appear to understand or communicates in very broken English, it is appropriate to ask what language the patient speaks at home and whether the patient can understand and speak English. In areas with large numbers of an ethnic minority, such as Spanish speakers, a practice should try to hire someone who speaks the language or train staff in the medical vocabulary of the target language. Children should not be used to translate except in emergencies because they may lack adequate vocabulary and understanding, and the patient may be reluctant to describe needs to a child. In some cases, an electronic translation device may be helpful, and some practices subscribe to telephone translation services. Commonly used instructions should be available in different languages. If the patient knows some English, using simple vocabulary and speaking slowly may help with comprehension.

Reviewing Insurance Card to Verify Coverage and Copayment

The patient's **insurance card** should be reviewed at the initial visit and the front (with plan information) and back (with contact information) copied and filed in the patient's medical record. Cards may vary somewhat but generally contain the name of the subscriber, which may be different from the name of the patient with family plans, as well as the ID number for the subscriber and the group. The plan code indicates the type of coverage. The patient's requirements regarding copayments are generally listed as well (front or back) and should be collected at the beginning or end of the visit.

```
Model Insurance
Subscriber:  Mary Jones
ID #:  ICU44444222286F
Group #:  777888226DM
Plan Code:  066

Office visit copay:    $25.00
ER copay:             $100.00

Verify ID.                  PPO
```

Coordination of Benefits and Birthday Rule

Coordination of benefits is the rules insurance companies use to ensure that no healthcare provider receives more than 100% of the charges submitted for services rendered. State regulations regarding coordination of benefits may vary somewhat, and some insurance policies have no coordination of benefits rules. If both spouses in a marriage have separate family insurance policies that cover spouse and/or children with coordination of benefits provisions, then the spouse whose birthday comes first in the year ("**birthday rule**") has the primary insurance and the other spouse, the secondary insurance. For those on Medicare but covered by an employer-provided insurance, the employer-provided insurance is primary and Medicare secondary. If, however, the Medicare recipient has only a Medigap (supplemental) insurance plan, then Medicare is primary. If parents are divorced, the parent the court has assigned as the responsible party has primary insurance. If there is no responsible party assigned, then a custodial parent who has remarried has the primary insurance. If the custodial parent has not remarried, then the birthday rule is in effect.

Tracer

The turn-around time for a claim submitted to an insurance company is usually 30 to 60 days if submitted on paper and 10 to 15 days if submitted electronically. Payments received after this time are considered delinquent. If a claim is delinquent, then the usual policy is to send a **tracer** within a few days to determine if there is a problem with the claim or if the insurance company requires more information. The insurance claim register should be checked routinely to ensure that delinquent claims are not overlooked. The tracer form should include:

- Name and address of insurance company.
- Patient's and insured's names.
- Employer's name (if appropriate).
- Date claim was initially submitted and the amount of the claim.
- Note indicating excess time has passed with no word from insurance company or request for further information.
- Area for the insurance company to explain reason for delay (pending, processing, denied).
- Physician's name, address, and telephone number.

Determining Appropriate Laboratory Tests for Patients

Patients often require **laboratory tests or imaging** that must be done in a different facility. Patients should not be referred to these facilities because the healthcare provider receives a financial benefit from doing so, such as payment for each referral or discounts, as this may be considered fraudulent under anti-kickback laws. State laws may vary, so the CMAA should be familiar with laws of the state he/she is practicing in. Whenever possible, patients should be given a choice of more than one facility and should be advised that they can choose where to go for testing. Patients should also be advised which facilities are in their network if the CMAA has this information or should be advised to check with their provider lists. In some areas, such as small towns, there may be only one option. In this case, patients should be so advised: "There is only one medical laboratory in town."

Insurance Terms

Terms Related to Insurance	
Cap	The protective strategy insurance companies utilize to limit the maximum dollar benefits for a policy. Caps may vary depending on the type of insurance. A routine accident and health benefits plan for one person may set a specific dollar maximum for that person, but a family plan may set a plan cap for the entire family and individual caps. Automobile insurance that covers bodily injury also usually has a category cap (such as $1 million for bodily injury) and per person caps (such as $250,000 per person), so one injured person cannot receive the entire amount.
Bundling	Occurs when an insurance plan negotiates a specific fee for a procedure, including all associated costs, and pays one bill.
Unbundling	Occurs when a bundled agreement is dissolved, and the insurance plan pays separate bills (hospital, anesthesiologist, surgeon, etc.).
Fee-for-service	The traditional billing method in which services are billed for separately.
Discounted fee-for-service	Similar to fee-for-service except that reimbursements are discounted.
Beneficiary	The person entitled to receive benefits.
Benefits	The amount the insurance company pays.
Dependent	Children and family members covered by a policyholder's insurance plan.
Eligibility	Refers to whether a person is entitled to benefits.
Exclusion	Items/Services for which benefits are not payable.
Guarantor	The person who is responsible for a bill (may be the same or different from the policyholder).
Policyholder	The person whose name is on the insurance policy and who (usually) pays for the plan.
Premium	The payment charged for an insurance policy.
Remittance advance	The Explanation of Benefits for Medicaid.
Rider	Special provision that expands or limits benefits.
Third-party payor	Person/Entity that pays a debt but was not involved in the contract that created the debt.

Credit Agreements

If patients are responsible for all or part of their bill for medical services and are not able to pay, the healthcare provider and the patient or guardian may draw up a **credit agreement**. The credit agreement includes the total amount owed and the payment schedule and amounts that have been agreed upon (usually monthly payments). If a patient simply notifies the healthcare provider of the intention to make payments and does so without discussing the matter with the healthcare provider, then no formal agreement is necessary. However, if the healthcare provider or staff discuss the matter with the patient/guardian and set up a schedule of payments, a formal written agreement is required. The credit agreement may include interest charges and charges for late payments. A truth-in-lending statement must be provided to the patient/guardian at the time the credit agreement is made.

#	Name	Filed	Amount	Current	31-60	61-90	91-120	120+	Balance total
1	T. Jones	2-10-19	$200.00	$200.00					$200.00
2	R. Moore	1-4-19	$100.00		$100.00				$100.00
3	M Snow	12-3-18	$480.00			$480.00			$480.00

Accounts Aging Record

The **accounts aging record** is used to track insurance payments, including those that are past due. The aging of accounts is done by 30-day increments (0-30, 31-60, etc.). Unless a payment agreement has been agreed upon in advance, all payments are considered past due after 30 days. Those that exceed 120 days are usually referred to a collection agency or written off by the practice. In some cases, the practice may send a letter asking for payment and indicating plans to take the matter to small claims court if payment is not received and the amount due is within the small claims court limits.

Coding Systems

ICD-10-CM and HCPCS Level II

International Classification of Diseases, 10th revision, Clinical Modifications, (ICD-10-CM) is a coding system used to code diagnoses. The ICD-10-CM codes are used for billing purposes to ensure that procedure codes match appropriate diagnoses. The codes all have at least 3 characters but may have up to 4 additional sub-categories. The first character must be alpha, the second and third, numeric, and the remaining alpha or numeric. A decimal point is placed after the first 3 characters. Diagnoses are classified by type of disease or system involved. For example, main categories include neoplasms and diseases of the respiratory systems. With ICD-10-CM, injuries are grouped by body part rather than category of injury. Thus, all injuries to the thorax (S20-S29) are grouped together. The chapter dealing with injuries, poisoning and other consequences of external causes are divided by two letters, S and T. The S-coded injuries are grouped by single body regions; however, some injuries are not localized, such as poisonings, and these are T-coded injuries.

CPT Codes

Current procedural terminology (CPT) codes were developed by the American Medical Association (AMA) and used to define those licensed to provide services and to describe medical and surgical treatments, diagnostics, and procedures. CPT 2012 codes specific procedures as well as typical times required for treatment. CPT codes are usually updated each October with revisions (additions, deletions) to coding. The use of CPT codes is mandated by both CMS and HIPAA to provide a uniform language and to aid research. These codes are used primarily for billing purposes for insurances (public and private). Under HIPAA, HHS has designed CPT codes as part of the national standard for electronic healthcare transactions:

- Category I codes are used to identify a procedure or service.
- Category II codes are used to identify performance measures, including diagnostic procedures.
- Category III codes identify temporary codes for technology and data collection.

HCPCS Level II Codes

Healthcare Common Procedure Coding Systems (HCPCS Level II) codes are used when filing claims for equipment, supplies and services that are not covered by CPT codes (Level I codes), including non-physician products such as durable medical equipment, ambulance services, laboratory service, orthotics, and prosthetics. HCPCS codes are also used for outpatient hospital care, chemotherapeutic drugs, and Medicaid:

- D codes are used for dental procedures.
- E codes are used for durable medical equipment, such as bedside commodes.
- L codes are used for orthotic and prosthetic procedures and devices, such as orthopedic shoes.
- P codes are used for pathology and laboratory services.

HCPCS Level II codes are comprised of 5 alphanumeric characters, beginning with a letter that indicates the grouping. For example, metal underarm crutches would be coded as E0114. The letter E indicates the item is durable medical equipment. The codes are updated on a quarterly basis.

Insurance Claim Register

An **insurance claim register** should be maintained either on paper or electronically to keep track of all insurance claims submitted and payments received, to ensure that claims are paid within the expected time limit so that follow-up can be carried out if necessary. While logs may vary, components often include:

- Claim number for the service provided.
- Patient's name
- Brief explanation of type of service and/or appropriate service code.
- Insurance carrier, ID and group number.
- Date and amount of the claim submitted.
- Date and amount of payment received.
- Difference between claim and payment.
- Follow-up date when further action is needed.
- Final disposition.

The register should be filled out after each claim is submitted; or, if claims are processed in bunches, the claims can be stacked and all entered into the register at the same time.

Tickler File

A **tickler file** is one that is used to hold copies of claim forms until receipt of payment. The file is arranged by months with separate dividers for each day of the month (1 through 31). When a claim is submitted, a copy of the claim form is placed in the tickler file under the date that is 6 weeks after the submission date, by which time payment should have been received. If payment has not been received by 6 weeks, then a follow-up letter should be sent to the insurance company and a notation of that made in the insurance claim register and the claim form and copy of the letter advanced an additional 2 to 6 weeks in the tickler file. The contents of the tickler file should be reviewed at the end of each billing period to determine if any submissions have not yet been paid or are overdue.

Medicare Options for Reimbursement

Under Medicare, healthcare providers have two **options for reimbursement**:

- Assignment of benefits: The healthcare provider agrees to accept Medicare payment as full-7payment for services covered by Medicare and payment is sent directly to the healthcare provider. Medicare pays 80% of customary and reasonable charges for the area (varies from one area to another). The healthcare provider cannot then submit a bill for the remaining 20% to the patient or secondary insurance and cannot bill the patients for additional charges. Healthcare providers may accept assignment for benefits for individual cases or for all patients. Healthcare providers must accept assignment for patients receiving both Medicare and Medicaid, for clinical laboratory services, ambulance services, drugs, and biologicals.
- Nonassignment of benefits: The healthcare provider does not agree to accept Medicare payments as payment in full so the patient submits a claim and directly receives reimbursement of 80% of customary and reasonable charges only. The patient (or secondary insurance) is responsible for additional charges.

Encounter Form

The **encounter form** contains CPT and ICD-10-CM codes and is used by the healthcare provider during visits to check off the correct type of visit and procedures as well as diagnoses. These then serve as the basis for billing. Each type of practice creates its own encounter form or uses a standardized form that corresponds. Because there are very many CPT and ICD-10-CM codes, one form cannot contain them all, so a practice chooses the codes that most apply to the procedures and diagnoses of that practice. For example, an orthopedic practice would include procedure codes for removing and applying a cast while a gynecological practice would include procedure codes for pelvic exams and pap smear and appropriate diagnostic codes.

Patient name:		File #:		Date:		Insurance:	
√	CPT code	Item	Fee	√	Diagnosis	ICD-10-CM code	
	99201	Minimal exam			Abd. Pain, unspec.	R10.9	
	99202	Focused exam			Abscess	L02	
	99203	Comp exam			Allergic reaction	T78.40	

Back Office Procedures

Patient Interviewing/History Taking Strategies and Techniques

Interviewing/History taking strategies and techniques include:

- Establishing rapport with the patient: Take time to make introductions and chat for a moment, especially if the patient appears anxious.
- Positioning within the patient's field of vision: Position in face-to-face position so that the patient does not have to look up or down during the interview.
- Avoiding medical jargon: Ask questions and respond in language that the patient is familiar with and explain any unclear terms used.
- Ensuring patient privacy/confidentiality: Be alert to the surroundings and make sure that questions and patient's responses remain confidential and cannot be overheard.

- Observing body language: Note non-verbal communication (eye contact, gestures, position, expressions, proxemics) for clues about the patient's emotional state and feelings.
- Asking open-ended questions: Avoid questions that can be answered with simple "yes" or "no" as much as possible.
- Allowing patient time to respond: Do not look at a watch, fidget, or appear in a hurry.
- Practicing active listening: Make eye contact, nod, respond, and pay attention when patient speaks.
- Respecting cultural differences: Avoid judgmental attitudes or comments.

SAMPLE Method of History Taking

SAMPLE Method of History Taking		
S	Signs and symptoms	Pain, bleeding, shortness of breath, injuries, fever, rash.
A	Allergies	Medications, environmental (foods, insects, plants, animals).
M	Medications	Prescribed, over-the-counter (OTC) vitamins/minerals, birth control and erectile dysfunction medications, herbal preparations, recreational drugs, other people's meds.
P	Past pertinent history	Especially related to current event.
L	Last oral intake	Foods, fluids, other substances.
E	Events (precipitating)	Occurrence just prior to event.

Injection Types, Locations, Angles, and Needle Sizes

Adult Injections			
Type	Gauge/ Needle	Angle	Sites
Intramuscular	19-25 g 1 or 1.5 to 3 inches	90°	(1) Upper outer arm (deltoid) for volumes of 0.5 to 2 mL, (2) upper outer hip (dorso-gluteal) for volumes of 1 to 3 mL (poses most risk of nerve injury and avoid with obese patients), (3) upper lateral hip (ventro-gluteal) for volumes 0.5 to 3 mL, (4) lateral middle third of thigh (vastus lateralis) for volumes of 0.5 to 3 mL.
Intradermal	27-28 g, 3/8 inch	15°	Inner surface of forearm, upper chest, upper back, back of upper arm. Volume <0.5 mL.
Subcutaneous	25-27 g, 3/8 to 5/8 inch	45-90°	Upper outer aspect of the arm (triceps area), the abdomen, the upper buttocks, and the upper outer aspect of the thigh. Volume to 1.5 mL.

Pulse Oximetry

Pulse oximetry utilizes an external oximeter that attaches to the patient's finger or earlobe to measure arterial oxygen saturation (SPO_2), the percentage of hemoglobin that is saturated with oxygen. The oximeter uses light waves to determine oxygen saturation (SPO_2). Oxygen saturation should be maintained >95% although some patients with chronic respiratory disorders, such as COPD may have lower SPO_2. Results may be compromised by impaired circulation, excessive light, poor positioning, and nail polish. If SPO_2 falls, the oximeter should be repositioned, as incorrect position is a common cause of inaccurate readings. Oximetry is used to monitor when patients are

- 36 -

on oxygen or mechanical ventilation. Oximeters do not provide information about carbon dioxide levels, so they cannot monitor carbon dioxide retention. Oximeters also cannot differentiate between different forms of hemoglobin, so if hemoglobin has picked up carbon monoxide, the oximeter will not recognize that.

Assessing Temperature

Temperature Assessment: Normal 37° C/98.6° F		
Oral (disposable)	1 to 3 minutes	Use only for children who can hold it under there tongue (≥4) but avoid with mouth breathers or those using oxygen. Eating, drinking, and smoking shortly before temperature assessment may affect results.
Oral (electronic)	10-60 seconds	Same as above. Most models beep when temperature reading is complete.
Axillary	10 minutes	Place under axilla and hold arm tightly against the thermometer. Normal is one degree F below oral temperature: 36.4° C /97.6° F.
Ear (electronic)	2 seconds	Point the tip toward the tympanic membrane (eardrum) for accuracy in reading. Waxy buildup in ear may interfere with results.
Rectal (glass)	3-5 minutes	Insert the thermometer gently into the rectum (do not force) about 1 inch and hold in place until temperature stops increasing. Remove promptly if the patient (usually an infant or small child) begins to struggle and risks breaking the thermometer or perforating the rectum. Normal is one-degree higher than oral temperature.
Rectal (electronic)	10-60 seconds	Same as above.

Assessing Normal Vital Signs from Neonate to Older Adulthood

Age	Heart rate	Respirations	BP (mm Hg)
Neonate (newborn)	100-220 (average 140-160) begins to slow after 3 months	40-60 for a few minutes, then 30-40	Systolic 70-90
Toddler (12-36 mo.)	80-130	20-30	Systolic 70-100
Pre-school (3 to 5)	80-120	20-30	Systolic 80-110
School-age (6-12)	70-110	20-30	80-120/60-80
Adolescence (13-18)	55-100	12-20	110-131/64-84
Early adulthood (19-40)	60-100 (average 80)	12-20	100-119/60-79 to 140/90 (high)
Mid. Adulthood (41-60)	60-100 (average 80)	12-20	100-119/60-79 to 140/90 (high)
Late adulthood (61+)	60-100 (average 70)	12-20	100-119/60-79 to 140/90 (high)

Assessing Pulse

Assessing Pulse	
Instructions: Pulse should be assessed with the 3rd and 4th fingers for one minute with light pressure to count the rate and determine if the pulse is regular or irregular. Pulse should not be assessed with the index finger because the CMAA may detect his/her own pulse rather than the patient's.	
Radial	Most commonly used site, located on the wrist above the thumb.
Temporal	On the side of the face about a half inch from the ear opening.
Carotid	On the right or left side of the throat beside the Adam's apple.
Apical	Left of the sternum at 4th intercostal space. Method of choice for infants and small children. May provide a more accurate reading for very irregular or weak adult pulses.
Brachial	At the inside of the elbow, inner aspect.
Femoral	On the right or left side of the groin, near the middle.
Popliteal	Behind the knee. Often used to assess circulation in the leg.
Dorsalis pedis	On the top of the foot, above the great toe.

Assessing Blood Pressure

Blood pressure can vary considerably. If an initial blood pressure is high, it should be retaken after a few minutes because it may be elevated because of patient anxiety ("white coat effect"). Using the correct blood pressure cuff size is essential for accuracy. The length of the bladder in the cuff should be equal to 80% of the arm's circumference, and the lower edge of the cuff when positioned should end about one inch above the antecubital fossa (inner elbow). For adults, inflate the cuff to 160 to 180 initially and increase pressure if pulse sounds are heard at that level. Usually, inflating the cuff to 100 to 120 initially is adequate for children. Extra-large cuffs are available for obese patients and pediatric cuffs for children. The BP is not usually assessed for infants. The CMAA can also palpate the brachial pulse while inflating the cuff; the systolic pressure is the point where the pulse is no longer palpable. At this point, the CMAA should continue inflating another 20 to 40 mm Hg and then begin deflating while auscultating. The first pulse heard is the systolic pressure; and the last heard, the diastolic pressure.

Specimen Labeling and Common Preservation Methods

Specimen Labeling

Before collecting a specimen, the patient's identity should be confirmed with two identifiers (name and birthdate). Every specimen container must have a label directly attached at the time and point of collection. The following information must be on each specimen: Patient's first and last name, medical record number, date of birth, date and time of collection, and initials of person collecting the sample. Infant samples also require the mother's first name, infant's gender, and infant's ID band number. Some labels may contain a barcode and/or the physician's name as well.

Preservation

Some specimens may be stored in the refrigerator, including urine and stool specimens, after being properly labeled. Fresh tissue specimens should be inserted into a container holding the fixative already with volume 20:1 in comparison with specimen. The container should be gently agitated for a few minutes after the specimen is inserted to ensure penetration.

Point-of Care Tests

Point of care tests may give qualitative results (present or absent, such as pregnancy test) or quantitative result (precise numbers, such as glucose). Quality control is critical in ensuring that test results are accurate and those performing the tests must be well-trained. Advantages include rapid turnaround time and small sample volumes. Additionally, a sample does not require pre-processing. Disadvantages include increased cost, quality variation, and billing concerns. Tests include:

- Glucose: A glucometer is used with a drop of blood from a finger obtained with a lancet and applied to a strip and inserted into the properly calibrated glucometer, which reports the results. Normal values for a child range from 60 to 100 mg/dL and for an adult under 100 mg/dL (fasting usually ranges from 70 to 100). Critical values are less than 40 g/dL or greater than 400 mg/dL. Non-glucose sugars, such as those in peritoneal dialysate can affect results.
- Coagulation: Point-of-care device uses a sample of whole blood to provide the patient's PT, aPTT, and INR for patients on warfarin anticoagulant. Some devices can measure activated clotting time (ACT) for patients on unfractionated heparin. For example, the CoaguChek X is a handheld meter used to monitor INR. A sample of capillary blood is obtained and a drop of blood placed on a test strip. The test strip must be inserted into the device within 15 seconds. Coagulation measurement begins and the results are displayed. Test results for these devices are comparable to standard testing. **INR:** (PT result/normal average): <2 for those not receiving anticoagulation and 2.0 to 3.0 those receiving anticoagulation. Critical value: >3-5 in patients receiving anticoagulation therapy.
- Pregnancy (human chorionic gonadotropin detection): Pregnancy tests are most accurate after a missed period and with the first morning urination. The patient should hold the testing stick in the stream of urine, or dip it in a cup of fresh urine. After the allotted wait time, the testing stick indicates whether the person is pregnant or not. False negatives may occur in early pregnancy.

Protocol for Needlestick Injury

If the CMAA experiences a **needlestick injury** while caring for a patient, the CMAA's initial response should be to wash the wound with soap and water. As soon as possible, the incident must be reported to a supervisor and steps taken according to established protocol. This may include testing and/or prophylaxis, depending on the patient's health history. In some cases, the patient may also be tested for communicable diseases, such as HIV, in order to determine the risk to the phlebotomist. PEP (post-exposure prophylaxis) is available for exposure to HIV (human immunodeficiency virus) and HBV (hepatitis B virus). However, no PEP is available for HCV (hepatitis C virus) although the CDC does provide a plan for management. PEP should be initiated within 72 hours of exposure. All testing and treatments associated with the needlestick injury must be provided free of cost to the CMAA.

Infection Control

Each medical practice should carry out a biological risk assessment each year or when new risks arise to determine the biosafety level and agent hazards and procedures hazards. Work practices should conform to Bloodborne Pathogen Standard (OSHA) and standard precautions (CDC). **Infection control** precautions include:

- Utilizing appropriate hand hygiene with hand-free sink for washing hands available near exit.
- Using mechanical pipettes instead of mouth pipetting.

- 39 -

- Eating, drinking, smoking, storing food, applying makeup, handling contact lenses all prohibited in the laboratory.
- Maintaining safe handling of sharps policies.
- Utilizing safety devices (retractable needles, lances) when possible.
- Minimizing splashing or aerosolizing liquids.
- Decontaminating potentially infectious materials prior to disposal.
- Packing potentially infectious materials for disposal outside of facility in appropriate packaging according to regulations.
- Maintaining a pest management program.
- Ensuring that all personnel are adequately trained.
- Ensuring appropriate immunizations and screening for personnel.
- Making PPE available and monitoring appropriate use.
- Ensuring eye wash station is easily accessed and available.

Hand Hygiene

The CMAA should carry out **hand hygiene** thoroughly with soap and water for one minute before working with patients and thereafter with soap and water (if hands are visibly soiled) or alcohol rub whenever the hands are contaminated, before applying gloves, before and after assisting patients, and after removing gloves. Antimicrobial soaps are only recommended if the hands have had contact with blood or body fluids. Note that any lotions applied to the hands should be compatible with latex. Jewelry and artificial nails should be avoided as they may harbor bacteria. Hand hygiene procedure:

- Wet hands thoroughly with warm water, apply soap, and rub hands together to massage the soap into the tissue, including between the fingers and about the nails.
- Rinse hands completely to remove all soap.
- Dry hands completely with clean towel or air dry.
- Use a clean towel or foot control to turn off the water.

If using alcohol rub, it should be thoroughly rubbed into all surfaces for at least 15 seconds. Drying time should take at least 15 seconds or insufficient rub was applied.

Preparing Daily Charts

Paper **charts** are generally pulled the evening before so that they are ready when the office first opens, based on the appointment schedule. Protocols vary from one practice to another depending on the preferences of the healthcare providers and the staff. The charts are usually organized in the order they will be seen. Once the charts are pulled, they should be assessed to determine that are complete and contain all recent reports. Charts should be started for new patients. An encounter form is usually filled out with the patient's name and placed on or in the charts. If electronic health records are used, then usually just the encounter forms are prepared as the charts will be accessed electronically although each file should be accessed before the appointment to make sure it is available and complete. The charts may be maintained at the front desk or other secure area so that the CMAA can place them outside the appropriate examining rooms. In some cases, healthcare providers prefer to have the charts placed on his/her desk so the healthcare provider can review them in advance.

Updating Patient's Charts with Progress Notes

Progress notes may take various forms (example is narrative), depending on the documentation format used although rules of documentation are essentially the same for all types. Military time is almost always used for documenting time so there is less chance of error in confusing AM and PM. No blank lines should be left that would allow later entries. Errors must be crossed out and "error" written. If a late entry is made, the date and time the entry was made should be entered and "Late entry" and the actual date and time of the event entered in parentheses (12-17-19, 11:45). Late entries should never be written above or between lines to try to fit it into the correct chronological order.

Date:	Time:	Progress notes:
02-05-19	13:30	Patient states she has had 2 episodes of palpitations lasting approximately 20 minutes in the past 3 days. She felt lightheaded at the times. --S. Brown, CMAA
02-17-19	12;45	~~Patient complaining of nausea persisting for 2 days.~~ --------------- Error --S. Brown, CMAA
02-17-19	14:40	Late entry (02-17-19, 11:45). Patient reports no further episodes of palpitations since starting metoprolol 25 mg BID. ----S. Brown, CMAA
03-12-19	15:00	Patient reports increasing muscle pain in legs since taking metoprolol. — (Continued on next page) --------------------S. Brown, CMAA

Office Logistics

Filing Systems

Alphabetic

When using an alphabetic filing system, records are filed according to the patient's last name in the following order:

Last name	First name	Middle initial (name)	Year of birth	Month of birth	Day of the month

If two or more patients have the same name, then the year of birth is the next item to consider with the earliest birth date filed first. Alphabetical filing is a simple method to understand and master, and it's relatively easy to retrieve records. However, if there are large numbers of patients, many people may have the same last and even first names, so retrieving files may become time-consuming. Additionally, last names fall disproportionately among a few letters (B, C, H, M, S, and W). One other problem is that this filing system gives no indication of when the patient was last seen, so reviewing records for this information would require each record be checked individually.

Indexing Rules

An initial is placed before a name beginning with the same letter	Brown, J. Brown, James
Ignore hyphens, apostrophes, and spaces	*Mary Kim-Mac Pherson* would be *Kimmacpherson, Mary.* Jake *O'Malley* would be *Omalley, Jake.*
If the surname of a foreign name is not clear, index as written	*Kim Seo-yeon* would be indexed as *Kim Seoyeon* (even though *Kim* is actually the surname)
Prefixes are considered part of the name	*De Koonig* would be indexed as Dekoonig
Commonly used abbreviated forms are included as used.	*St. Germaine* would be indexed as *Stgermaine.*
Titles without a surname are considered the first unit for indexing.	*Sister Marie* would be indexed as *Sistermarie.*
Articles are disregarded	*The Healing Clinic* would be indexed as *Healingclinic (the).*

Numeric

When using a **numeric filing system**, records are filed according to an assigned number. Approaches include:

- Direct numeric: Numbers are assigned in ascending numeric order to patients. Files easy to retrieve, but a master patient index (with patients listed alphabetically) must be accessed first to obtain the patient's file number. For small practices, this method may take more time than an alphabetical filing system; but for large practices, it may be more efficient.
- Terminal digit: Numbers are assigned in 3 parts. For a record numbered 44-62-10, the record will be filed in section 10 as the last digits are the primary set of numbers referred to for filing purposes, and the middle set (62) is the secondary set, indicating the correct subsection in section 10. The chart will be placed between in section 10, in subsection 62 and between records 43 and 45. This filing method is one of the most efficient when there are large numbers of records.

- Middle-digit: Similar to terminal digit, but the middle digit is the primary set of numbers, followed by the first digits and then the last. For example, 22-17-24 would be filed in section 17, shelf number 22, and folder 24.

Alphanumeric, Year of Birth, and Family Filing

A number of different **filing systems** are in use, some developed to meet the specific needs of a practice:

- Alphanumeric: A number is assigned to each patient (as with numeric filing) and a master index file created to access the number, but each number is preceded by the first two or three letters of the patient's last name. For example, Mary Bradley may be assigned the number BRA788.
- Year of birth: In this system, files are places in sections corresponding to their birth dates according to this order:

| Year of birth | Month | Day | Last name | First name | Middle initial |

Year of birth filing may be used in practices where the patient's age is an important factor, such as in a mammography center.

- Family filing: All members of a family are filed under the primary caregiver's name (often the mother). This filing practice in common in pediatric practices.

Electronic

Electronic health records may be stored onsite or in the cloud in secured and encrypted databases. For onsite storage, servers should be maintained in locked, climate-controlled rooms with servers rack-mounted and regular surveillance. Vulnerable devices should remain in the locked room. Data should be backup up routinely and stored/archived in a secure remote location. Cloud storage is managed by a third-party service provider although the services provided may vary. For patient records, each patient is assigned a patient identifying number and the records may be accessed by various fields, including the ID number, the patient's name, or birthdate. Access is password protected. In some cases, print documents and images are scanned into the electronic health record, but in other cases, the print documents and images are maintained in separate paper files, making retrieval of the patient's records more time-consuming and increasing the risk of errors (such as lost or misplaced documents).

Cross-Referencing of Medical Records

Cross-referencing is providing a notation in one place that directs to another place. Cross-referencing may refer to information inside one record or to information in different records. Cross-referencing is especially important in being able to quickly access medical records. For example, if a patient is married and uses her maiden name (Marion Clark) for business purposes but uses a hyphenated form of her spouse's and her last name (Marion Clark-Jones) or simply her spouse's last name for other purposes, the primary file may be listed as Marion Clark-Jones but cross-referenced as Marion Clark and Marion Jones. Cross referencing may be necessary if a patient, for example, has an ethnic legal name such as Jae-Seong Park but goes by the name Jason Park. Steps to cross-referencing include:

- Determine the primary listing and create a record where all medical records should be placed.
- Identify various alternatives names by which the file might be located.
- Create a cross-reference sheet or insert (such as a piece of cardstock with cross reference information on it) to be placed in the files.

EHR/EMR

The **electronic health/medical record** (EHR/EMR) is a digital computerized patient record that may be integrated with CPOE and CDSS to improve patient care and reduce medical error. Software applications vary considerably, and standardization has not yet been implemented, so each organization must carefully review current and future anticipated needs as well as the ability of applications to interface with each other to provide for adequate measurements, data collection, reports, retrieval of data, analysis, and confidentiality. Increasingly, physicians in private practice, especially those in large groups, are employing EHRs, which may be different systems than those used in hospitals. Systems can be customized to meet the needs of the organization, but cost and lack of standardization remain barriers for implementation. However, studies indicate that there is a positive correlation between comprehensive EHR systems and patient outcomes. Quantifiable data about cost-effectiveness can be difficult to calculate because savings are often in terms of saved time, fewer interventions, and reduced error.

Personal Health Record

Elements

Personal health records (PHR) are electronic records that include information for the electronic health record generated by healthcare providers as well as information provided by the individual patient, allowing the patient to access, record, and share health information. Many different applications exist for creating a PHR. Elements of a PHR should include:

- The individual has the ability to control the PHR.
- The information in the PHR is comprehensive and covers the patient's lifetime.
- The information in the PHR derives from all healthcare providers.
- The PHR can be easily accessible at any time from any location with access.
- The information contained in the PHR is secure and cannot be accessed without proper authorization.
- The PHR discloses who entered data and when as well as who has accessed the data.
- Exchange of information with different healthcare providers across the healthcare system is efficient.
- PHRs should help to deliver care more cost-effectively and efficiently.

Types

Paper/ Personal files	Patient-maintained paper records can include booklets, files, notebooks, medication records, and handwritten notations. While data can be aggregated from various sources, this method is time consuming, quality varies widely, and data cannot always be easily or quickly retrieved.
Non-tethered	Non-tethered PHRs are stand-alone and not connected to a particular system or EHR. Information may be carried on a smart card, flash card, CD, or DVD. These pose more security risks than tethered PHRs and require more input from the individual to maintain accurate records.
Tethered	Data are tied to a particular system and EHR and are often web-based. A secure patient portal is provided so the individual can access all or parts of the records, including lists of medications and laboratory results. Examples include Kaiser's HealthConnect and the VA's My HealthVet. Interactivity varies but may include health diaries and logs.
Networked	Data is derived from multiple sources in a network rather than one system. This allows for more flexibility.

Patient Use

The **personal health record** (PHR) presents an opportunity for patient participation in healthcare care in a number of ways:

- Data entry: Most PHRs allow patients to enter some types of data, although this may vary. Typical data entry includes personal and family health history, use of complementary therapy, and health behaviors (such as diet and exercise). Some also allow entry of health data, such as BP readings, daily BS, and weight.
- Delegation: PHRs usually allow the patient to assign a delegate or proxy (such as a caregiver or immediate family member) to access the PHR. In most systems, parents can access information for a child until age 13 but the child may assign a parent as proxy after that age although selected information (such as sexual history, treatment) may be blocked.
- Messaging: Many systems allow patients to send secure messages to healthcare providers, in some cases routing them through a triage team.

Data Entry Procedures

Data entry procedures include posting:

- Charges: If the physician/nurse practitioner manually checks off services, print out a charge slip from the computer program and later use the information on the form to enter data into the computer application. In the charge posting screen, post the patient's name, identification number, date of service, the service provided (office visit, ECG, injection), the CPT code, the ICD-10-CM diagnostic codes, HCPCS Level II codes, and the charge for the service. The application may require co-payments and payments to be entered as well. Diagnostic codes much match the service provided.
- Payments: Access the payment posting screen, which should list the procedure charge history, and post the correct date, payment type (cash, check, credit card), and amount, and check the balance (view ledger).
- Adjustments: Discounts, such as for Medicare or insurance, are usually entered in the charge posting screen, but this may vary from one application to another. The adjustment is to the balance owed.

Medical Records

Source-Oriented

With **source-oriented medical records**, each type of service has a different section with information in each section organized with the latest on top so it is first accessed. This is the most traditional form of medical record information utilized in hospitals, and often utilized narrative documentation:

- Demographic: Basic identifying information, such as name, age, contact information, and insurance information.
- Progress notes: Placed next because they are accessed most frequently.
- History and physical examination.
- Laboratory reports.
- Imaging reports and other non-laboratory diagnostic test reports.
- Consultation reports.
- Other reports, such as from hospitalization, PT, OT, speech therapy, rehabilitation, recreational therapy.
- Correspondence of any type.
- Other non-treatment documents, such as living wills, transfer forms, preauthorization forms.

Problem-Oriented Organization

With **problem-oriented medical records**, records are arranged according to a problem list. This format is often used with electronic health records and is currently the most common organization. The medical record is typically divided into four different sections:

- Database: All reports regarding the patient's physical status are filed in this section, including all laboratory, imaging, and other diagnostic reports and history and physical exam.
- Problem list: Current and past problems are dated, listed, and numbered. This section includes lists of medications, list of allergies, and immunization history. The problem list is followed when assessing a patient to ensure that all issues are addressed routinely and not overlooked. Some problems may be resolved and others may be added to the list.
- Plan of treatment: This section includes physician's orders regarding treatment, diagnostic tests, referrals and the need for follow-up. In some cases, this section may be simply included in the progress note section.
- Progress notes: Each problem is addressed by number, usually in the SOAP format. Flowcharts are often used to document problems.

Collection of Copayments and Receipt for Payment

During check-in procedures, the patients' insurance information should be collected and any required **copayment** noted. The patient is usually asked to pay the copayment prior to being seen by a healthcare provider although some practices may collect the copayment at the end of service. A good approach is "How would you like to make your $20 copayment?" Credit card payment usually provides a print receipt, but the CMAA should provide a payment receipt for all cash payments.

Those paying with a check usually consider the cancelled check an adequate receipt and may not want a printed receipt. The payment receipt is usually a simple form.

Jones Medical Practice
Date: _____

Received from _____ Amount $ _____

For _____

Check _____ Cash _____ Credit card _____ Money Order _____

Received by _____

Financial Procedures

Invoices and Pre-Invoices

Invoices are essentially billing forms that describe a purchase/service and the amount due to pay for the purchase/service. Invoices include the patient's name, account number, a brief description of the purchase or service provided, the charge, any payment received, and the balance due as well as the date by which the payment is due. Invoices are generally sent by mail and may include a return envelope to facilitate payment. Invoices are usually mailed on a regularly scheduled basis, such as on the 15th and last day of the month. Payment is usually due within 2 to 4 weeks. **Pre-invoices** are estimates of charges. For example, patients scheduled for procedures may receive pre-invoices that list the scheduled services and the estimated charges for each service.

Indigent Patients

Some patients are **indigent** and lack insurance and cannot afford to pay for healthcare. If patients present with no insurance, the CMAA should ask how they plan to pay and if they indicate in advance that they cannot, options include:

- Refer to social services to determine if they are eligible for Medicaid.
- Explore reasons for illness/injury to determine if they are eligible for Worker's Compensation or payment through an automobile insurance.
- Refer to a public hospital or emergency department that provides care to those without funds.
- Arrange a payment plan that allows them to pay what they can afford each month.
- Provide service free of charge.

In some cases, patients may intend to pay but later find themselves without adequate funds and are unable to pay. In these cases, options include writing off the entire debt or lowering the fee. If lowering the fee, for example from $200 to $50, the bill should continue to be for $200 until the $50 is paid and then the remaining $150 written off.

Overdue Bills

If a patient has not paid an **overdue bill**, the CMAA may telephone the patient after a specified period of time (usually over 30 days). Before telephoning, the CMAA should gather information about the outstanding bill and any insurance. The CMAA should remain courteous and respectful during the call and avoid demanding payment and should make the call in private between 8 AM and 9 PM. Before discussing the matter, the CMAA must verify the identity of the person answering the phone and should use the person's complete name, "Is this Mary C. Smith?" Subsequent steps include:

1. Ask if the patient has time to talk or agree to a later time to call.
2. Explain the purpose of the call without making apologies, "This is Dr. Jones's medical assistant Sarah Brown. I'm calling about your account."
3. Explain that the account is overdue and try to schedule payments by a specified date.
4. If no payment is again received, telephone again.
5. If no payment is received within 90 to 120 days, a final statement asking for payment must be sent before the account can be turned over to a collection agency.

Skips

In some cases, patients move without leaving a forwarding address (purposefully or accidentally) and bills are returned without a forwarding address (**"skips"**). Steps include:

1. Try to telephone the patients as they may have kept the same telephone numbers.
2. Call any third-party references on the patients' medical records and discreetly ask how to locate the patients without explaining why. Note it is illegal to contact a third party for such information more than one time unless the third party specifically asks for another contact ("Call me in a week"). Document all contacts and their responses.
3. Search the Internet for information about the person, including social media sites such as Facebook.
4. Search on a people search site, such as PeopleSearch or TruthFinder. These sites charge a fee for information.
5. Turn account over to a collection agency if unable to locate the patients.

Petty Cash

Petty cash is a small amount of cash (usually no more than $100) that is kept on hand to pay for miscellaneous costs, such as for overdue postage, tips for delivery, parking costs, and supplies, such as coffee or tea, for a break room. Petty cash should be kept in a locked, secure drawer or container. Money placed into petty cash should come from a practice account but never directly from cash payments directly received from a patient. That money should be kept separate. A petty cash record should be maintained and should include a record of any disbursement and replenishment. The date and purpose of disbursements must be recorded along with the signature of the person withdrawing funds. Additionally, petty cash receipts should be filled out each time a person receives money from petty cash, such as when a person withdraws money to purchase breakroom supplies.

Bookkeeping

Single Entry

With **single-entry bookkeeping**, only one entry is made for each transaction. This is a simple form of bookkeeping, similar to maintaining records in a checkbook, so minimal training is required of staff involved in financial record keeping. Single-entry bookkeeping may vary somewhat. For example, if set up to record copayments, the record may only have entries for income, but a typical single-entry system would record both income and expenses.

Date	Description	Ref #	Income	Expense	Balance
Jan. 1	Balance				500.00
Jan 12	Printer cartridges	1		126.00	374.00
Jan. 15	Vitamin supplements	2	50.00		424.00
Jan. 16	Cash deposit	3	20.00		474.00

Double Entry

With **double-entry bookkeeping,** each transaction requires two entries: a debit, which shows a decrease in assets (liabilities plus owner's equity), and a credit, which shows an increase in equities (net worth). Debits are entered on the right side of a ledger and credits on the left. Total debits should be equal to total credits. Double-entry bookkeeping is the most commonly used form of bookkeeping for large businesses and organizations. For assets, inflows are posted under debits and outflows under credit, but for liabilities inflows are posted under credits and outflows under debits. With double-entry bookkeeping, for example, a payment received from an insurance company to pay for services provided to a patient would be entered as a credit in assets because it increases the total value of the practice, but it would be entered as a debit in liabilities because it decreases the amount of money that the practice owes. Double-entry bookkeeping generally must be managed by an accountant.

Pegboard or "Write It Once"

A **pegboard or "write-it-once"** form of record keeping is used in many medical offices, even those with computerized records (as a backup). With this form of record keeping, a pegboard (pegs on the left side of a flat writing board) is used to hold a number of different documents (day sheet, patient ledger, receipt/superbill) stacked one on top of the other. When data is entered by ballpoint pen into the top document, it transfers through non-carbon coatings to the underlying documents so that these documents do not need to be filled out separately and the patient and/or CMAA is required to sign only one time. This can save considerable time and reduce the chance of error. It's important to make sure documents are properly aligned and that adequate pressure is exerted when entering data.

Bookkeeping Terminology

Accounts receivable	Money owed to a practice/business after products have been delivered or services provided. Payment is usually expected within 30 days.
Accounts payable	Money that a practice/business owes to creditors, such as vendors or banks. Payments must be made in accordance to the contract or agreement to avoid late payment fees.
Adjustment	Entry made into a ledger to change an account, such as by entering a discount.
Assets	Liabilities plus owner's equity.
Day sheet	Record of daily transactions.
Disbursement	Money that is paid out for expenses.
Expenses	Money needed to pay for running a practice/business.
Liabilities	Net worth (debts, income, customer deposits and prepayments).
Owner's equity	Assets of a practice/business minus liabilities.

Posting	Transferring information from one type of record to another.
Received on account	Partial payment for a debt owed to the practice/business.
Revenue	Money received as payment.

Handling Mail

Incoming **mail** should be sorted and distributed according to a protocol established for the office. Typically, mail addressed directly to a healthcare provider or marked as "personal" or "confidential" is placed in that person's box but mail addressed to the practice is placed in the medical director or manager's box. Mail from vendors usually goes to the medical director/manager. Mail from insurance companies is routed to the person responsible for insurance. Whether the CMAA opens mail or not and the types of mail the CMAA opens varies from one practice to another. When packages are received, they should be opened, the packing receipts retrieved and the contents checked against the packing receipt to ensure that all items were shipped and arrived intact. Any missing or damaged items or notices of backorder must be noted and reported to the sender.

Day Sheet

A **day sheet** is a record of daily transactions (procedures, charges, income, adjustments, expenses, and balances) for each day of practice. Day sheets may vary in complexity from simple to more complex and may be completed on a paper form or a computerized form. Income is usually recorded when it is received rather than billed, and bills are recorded when they are paid rather than received. All patients' names may be recorded on the day sheet along with previous balances at the beginning of the day (although this may result in blank lines if patients cancel), or the names can be added as patients arrive. Payments that arrive in the mail or through automatic deposit are recorded on the day sheet as they are received. The day sheet may be completed with information derived from the charge slip, superbill, and ledger.

Mail Options

First class	Mail delivery for items weighing 12 ounces or less. Usually the fastest method of delivery because of automated sorting.
Certified	USPS service for first class mail/packages or Priority mail. Sender receives a receipt and receiver must sign to receive mail/package. Tracking available. Proof of delivery maintained for 2 years by USPS. Return Receipt (proof of delivery) can be purchased. May take up to 5 days for delivery.
Registered	Similar to certified but transported per locked or sealed containers and tracking available. Insurance can be purchased for up to $25,000. May take up to 15 days for delivery.
Priority	Mail delivery for items weighing 13 ounces to 70 pounds. Tracking and insurance available. Flat rate packages are available. Must be sorted manually so usually slower than first class.
USPS Priority mail express	Expedited mail delivery with guaranteed overnight, 1-3 days delivery, 2-3 days delivery (only packages), or 2-8 days delivery.
USPS Retail ground	Mail delivery for items over 70 pounds and up to 130 inches of length/girth combined. Delivery may be slower than priority mail.
USPS Media Mail	Low-cost option for media and educational materials weighing no more than 70 pounds.

FedEx	Non-governmental courier service that provides international shipping. Guaranteed delivery times available for most shipments. Insurance available. One rate pricing available for envelopes weighing less than 10 pounds and packages weighing less than 50 pounds. Handles packages of 3 to 150 pounds. Offers tracking and Saturday delivery.
UPS & DHL	Services similar to FedEx. DHL is based in Germany rather than the US. Both provide Saturday delivery.

Compliance

Ensuring Security of Electronic Applications Containing Patient Information

Measures to ensure the **security of electronic applications** containing patient information include:

- Password: Passwords should be strong but not so complex that users write them down because that increases risk of unauthorized access. Passwords should be changed on a regularly scheduled basis, such as monthly. Passwords should not be birthdates, anniversary dates, or names of children or pets.
- Screen saver: Medical screensavers should be set to automatically launch after a specified period of time to protect any information that may be left on the screen.
- Encryption: All information entered into the application or transmitted must be encrypted (protected by converting to code) so that it cannot be accessed without the proper password.
- Firewall: A computer application or hardware that blocks unauthorized access to computer programs and data and monitors incoming data to ensure its safety. Firewalls can also block Internet users from accessing private networks (such as medical networks).

Breach Notification

HIPAA Breach Notification Rule requires covered entities to report any breaches in protected health information:

- Individuals: Notification by standard mail or email (if the individual has agreed) as soon as possible but no later than 60 days after the breach. If lacking contact information for 10 or more individuals, notice must be placed on the organization's website for 90 days with a tollfree telephone number or notice provided in print or broadcast media. For fewer than 10 individuals, alternate notification, such as by telephone, is permitted. Individual breaches are reported to the HHS Secretary annually.
- 500 or more individuals: In addition to individual notification, notice must be given in prominent media outlet serving the affected states no later than 60 days after the breach. The HHS Secretary must be notified electronically within 60 days after the breach. If the breach affected fewer than 500 individuals, the HHS Secretary must be notified within 60 days of the end of the calendar year in which the breaches occurred.

HIPAA-Compliant Sign-in Sheets

Sign-in sheets are covered by the HIPAA Privacy Rule and are allowed to contain the following information:

- Date and arrival time.
- Patient's name.
- Time of the appointment.
- Healthcare provider's name.

Any other information included must in no way be identifying. The sign-in sheet cannot contain any information about the reason for the appointment, such as "blood pressure check" as others signing in would be privy to this health information. The CMAA can use the information in the sign-in sheet

- 52 -

when calling for the patient: "Ms. Brown, Dr. Jones can see you now." Some practices use initials for sign-in sheets instead of names, especially in practices dealing with sensitive diagnoses, such as STDs or HIV/AIDS. If more information is desired on a sign-in sheet, such as the name of a test they are scheduled for, then separate sign-in sheets can be given to patients to fill out and hand in, but they should not be left where others could read them.

#	Name	Appt time	Arrival time	Appt. with	New (√)
1	Terry Jamison	8:30	8:20	Dr. Stephens	
2	M.J. MALEK	9:00	8:55	DR. STEPHENS	√
3	Lucy Madsen	9:00	8:45	Dr. Rubin	

Public Health Statutes Related to Public Health and Welfare Disclosure

Public health statutes related to public health and welfare disclosure include:

- Communicable diseases: Title 42 (The Public Health and Welfare) and each state's regulations control reporting requirements for communicable diseases and for quarantine. Diseases that must be reported to the CDC include cholera, giardiasis, hepatitis, salmonellosis, shigellosis, and cryptosporidiosis. State requirements vary, but generally include influenza and measles.
- Vital statistics: Each state has a department of vital statistics that compiles birth and death records.
- Abuse/Neglect against children/older adults: All states have laws regarding abuse/neglect, and all healthcare providers are mandatory reporters. Reporting agencies may differ from one state to another.
- Wounds of violence: All states have laws regarding which types of wounds of violence (usually knife and gunshot wounds) that must be reported to the police.

Authorization for Release of Medical Information

Before medical records can be released, the patient or an authorized representative must sign an **authorization for release of medical records**. While formats vary widely, the form must state explicitly which records (all records, specific records) that are to be released and to whom. Patients have the right to write in any restrictions to sharing of information that they want. Sharing information that is not covered by the release is a HIPAA violation although a power of attorney gives another individual the right to request information, and records may be legally be released upon receiving a subpoena for the records. Generally, parents/legal guardians can request records of minors except (1) where the state gives minors the right to consent to certain types of care, (2)

- 53 -

when the court has authorized care of a minor, and (3) when the physician, patient, and parent/guardian have all agreed that the care provided by the physician will be confidential.

```
┌─────────────────────────────────────────────────────────────────────┐
│              Authorization for Release of Medical Records             │
│                        Jones Medical Practice                         │
│                             224 X Street                              │
│                            San Jose, CA                              │
│                                                                       │
│  Patient's name _____   Date of birth _____  Last 4 digits SS# _____ │
│                                                                       │
│  Address: _____  City _____  State _____           │
│                                                                       │
│  Phone # _____                                             │
│                                                                       │
│  I hereby authorize and request Jones Medical Practice to release by ____ Mail ___ Fax ___ Secure email │
│                                                                       │
│  Protected health information including ____ All records OR ____ Specific items only (list below) │
│  _____  │
│                                                                       │
│  to: Name _____  Address _____     │
│                                                                       │
│  Phone # _____  Fax # _____  Email _____       │
│                                                                       │
│  Signature (Patient or authorized representative) _____  Date _____ │
│                                                                       │
│  Witness signature _____  Date _____                    │
└─────────────────────────────────────────────────────────────────────┘
```

Penalties for HIPAA Violations

In order to remain in compliance with HIPAA regulations, an organization must carry out 6 annual audits: security risk, privacy, HITECH Subtitle D, security standards, asset and device, and physical sit. All Staff members must have annual training regarding HIPAA and security awareness training. Identity management and control of access must be in place and access to electronic PHI monitored. Patients must receive a Notice of Privacy Practices.

Category	Circumstances	Fine
1	The entity was not, and could not reasonably have been expected to be, aware of the violation.	$100 to $50,000 per violation.
2	The entity knew, or should reasonably have known, about the violation, but did not "act with willful neglect."	$1,000 to $50,000 per violation.
3	The entity "acted with willful neglect," but corrected it swiftly (within 30 days) once they became aware of the violation.	$10,000 to $50,000 per violation
4	The entity "acted with willful neglect" and failed to correct the violation in a timely manner.	$50,000 per violation

An organization may be fined up to $1.5M per calendar year for all identical violations of a given HIPAA provision. Violations of multiple provisions increase the annual cap linearly.

Criminal Penalties/Employee Sanctions

HIPAA violations may result in not only civil penalties but also jail or prison terms, depending on the type of violation and mitigating factors. Lack of knowledge of HIPAA rules and regulations is not considered justification for violations:

- Criminal penalties:
  - Tier 1: Reasonable cause or the entity had no knowledge of the violation—up to one year of incarceration.
  - Tier 2: Protected health information obtained under false pretenses—up to 5 years of incarceration.
  - Tier 3: Protected health information obtained and used for personal profit or for malicious purpose—up to 10 years of incarceration.
- Employee sanction: May result from action on the part of the employee or even for failing to report a HIPAA violation by another employee (such as unauthorized access of a patient's medical records). Sanctions may vary according to the organization and the type of violation but may include suspension, termination of employment, or loss of licensure.

Passwords

Passwords, which are usually used with a username and are used to access protected data, should be changed every 30 to 60 days. More frequent changes make it hard for people to remember their passwords, so they are more likely to write them down, increasing the risk of security breaches. Strong passwords include combinations of letters (capital and lower case), numbers, and symbols/signs, such as the ampersand (&) and are harder to break than dictionary words. Users should never share passwords. Tokens are items used to authenticate a person's identity and allow access to a system. They commonly require the use of not only the token but also a PIN or user name and password. Tokens may be in the form of access cards, which may utilize different technologies: Photos, optical-coding, electric circuits, and magnetic strips. They may also be contained in common objects, such as a key fob. Some tokens must be plugged directly into the computer. Different types of tokens include: ID cards, challenge-response tokens, and smart cards.

Peer-to-Peer Information

With access to the Internet, **peer-to-peer information** has taken on new importance. A message board or website is available online for virtually every condition and disease. On these sites, patients and family members can often share experiences and give advice to each other. Patients may hear about new or different treatment approaches or medications and call or visit to ask for changes in their plans of care. One problem is that what works for one patient may not work for another, and since the people on the sites often lack a medical background, their information may be inaccurate. However, people may derive many benefits, including not only information but emotional support. Some, such as *Smart Patients*, host multiple "communities" related to diseases and have links to research articles and clinical trials. With knowledge, patients and families have a better understanding of their rights and the options available to them.

Appropriate Discussion of Patients' Medical Information

Discussions of patients' medical information should be restricted to the facility and carried out only with those who are authorized to obtain information about the patients, such as the healthcare provider and nurses directly caring for the patient. Discussions about patients' care or issues should never be discussed in any public venue or where unauthorized people may overhear. For example, discussions should not take place at the front desk where waiting patients and family may overhear and should never take place in a cafeteria, even if it's in the healthcare facility. If the CMAA is present and overhears others discussing patients, the CMAA should intervene and point out that their discussion was overheard and that they are violating the patients' rights. If they are resistant, then pointing out that they could lose their jobs may help to make the point.

Legal Implications

Patient Data Misuse

Patient data misuse is an increasing problem with the rapid proliferation of EHRs. Types of misuse include:

- Identity theft: Someone obtains identifying information, such as Social Security numbers and credit card numbers as well as birthdates and addresses, for fraudulent purposes.
- Unauthorized access: Although EHRs and computerized documentation systems are password protected, providers sometimes share passwords or unwittingly expose their passwords to others when logging in, allowing others to access information about patients.
- Privacy violations: Even those authorized to access a patient's record may share private information with others, such as family or friends.
- Security breach: Data is vulnerable to security breach because of careless of inadequate security, especially when various business associates, such as billing companies, have access to private information.

Privacy and Security Rules

HIPAA mandates **privacy and security rules** (CFR, Title 45, part 164) to ensure that health information and individual privacy is protected:

- Privacy rule: Protected information includes any information included in the medical record (electronic or paper), conversations between the doctor and other healthcare providers, billing information, and any other form of health information. Procedures must be in place to limit access and disclosures.
- Security rule: Any electronic health information must be secure and protected against threats, hazards, or non-permitted disclosures, in compliance with established standards. Implementation specifications must be addressed for any adopted standards. Administrative, physical, and technical safeguards must be in place as well as policies and procedures to comply with standards. Security requirements include: limiting access to those authorized, use of unique identifiers for each user, automatic logoff, encryption and decryption of protected healthcare information, authentication that healthcare data has not been altered/destroyed, monitoring of logins, authentication, and security of transmission. Access controls must include unique identifier, procedure to access system in emergencies, time out, and encryption/decryption.

Mandatory Reporting

While laws about **mandatory reporting** vary from state to state, healthcare providers, including medical assistant personnel, are considered mandatory reporters in all states and must report suspected cases of child and elder abuse and neglect. The CMAA must follow state guidelines for reporting as simply notify the receiving facility of suspected child abuse is not adequate. The CMAA should be familiar with the signs of abuse and neglect (certain types of fractures, unexplained or multiple bruises, suspicious bruise patterns, burns, hair loss, and inadequate food, clothing, shelter). Additionally, in most states certain types of injuries or assaults must be reported to law enforcement, including stab wounds, gunshot wounds, and sexual assaults. Each state has lists of

- 56 -

specific communicable diseases (such as TB and measles) that must be reported—some required by the CDC but others specific to the state or local area. Those classified as urgent (such as Ebola) must be reported immediately while others may be reported within one to seven working days. Reporting procedures vary.

System Security and Integrity

Device Access Control

Device access control can encompass a wide range of technologies and procedures. The first step is to determine what classes of users have access to different devices and then what method of authentication (password, biometrics) for role and entity-based access is required. Clear policies and procedures must be in place for both access and use of devices. Role and entity-based access should be determined by the individual role and function within the organization rather than on hierarchy. Networked medical devices and information technology (IT) devices may be on the same network and handheld devices may connect to multiple networks, so these situations pose additional security risks. All handheld devices, which pose the most risk, must be password protected. Security of access control must be strictly enforced and those who violate security policies and procedures should have use restricted. Each potential user of devices must be correctly identified and access controlled. Commercial access control programs are available for healthcare organizations.

Time-Out

Once a person has logged in and gained access to a computer, the computer is vulnerable if that user leaves the computer and fails to log out, so computers connected to a secure system routinely have a **time-out** feature (automatic log off) that locks the system after a prescribed period (usually 10 to 15 minutes) in which there is no mouse or keyboard activity. Some software programs and applications also have time-out features. Once the time out is initiated, a person must log in again in the prescribed manner to gain access. Time out/Automatic logoff is one of the security procedures that must be addressed for part of HIPAA's security rule. The users' workflow and type of use of devices should be considered when scheduling automatic log off. Computer screens must be situated so that they cannot be observed by those who are unauthorized.

OSHA

Infection Control

The **Occupational Safety and Health Administration** (OSHA) requires that safeguards to prevent occupational exposure and incidents be a part of infection control policies. Additionally, the FDA has requirements related to the safety of medical devices. Some states have regulations that are more restrictive than those of OSHA. Important elements include:

- An exposure control plan that outlines methods to reduce staff injury/ exposure.
- Use of universal precautions at all times with all individuals.
- Planning work practices to minimize danger and using newer and safer technologies as they become available, such as needles engineered to prevent injury.
- Sharps disposal methods that prohibit bending, recapping, shearing, breaking, or handling contaminated needles or other sharps. Scooping with one hand may be used if recapping is essential.
- Workers must be trained in use of universal precautions and methods to decrease exposure.

- Procedures for post-exposure evaluation and treatment must be part of exposure control plan.
- Immunization with Hepatitis B vaccine available to healthcare workers.

Role

The **Occupational Safety and Health Administration** (OSHA) is part of the Department of Labor and is charged with ensuring safe, healthful working condition and setting and enforcing workplace standards. OSHA covers most employers in the private sector, but state and federal safety regulations also generally conform to OSHA standards. Employers must provide safety training, must inform workers of chemical hazards, and must provide required personal protective equipment. OSHA must be notified of a workplace-related death within 8 hours and workplace-related injury that results in hospitalization, loss of eye, or amputation within 24 hours. Workers may file a complaint about workplace conditions with OSHA and request an inspection. OSHA whistleblower program prohibits retaliation. OSHA provides HAZWOPER training courses (8-hour, 24-hour, 40-hour, and refresher) for first responders. OSHA has established regulations and guidelines that are industry specific. For example, OSHA has regulations regarding emergency medical services. OSHA requires hazardous material be color-coded with red indicating danger; yellow, caution; orange, warning; and fluorescent orange/orange-red, biological hazard.

Reporting Forms

OSHA provides 3 basic forms to report work-related injuries, which is any injury resulting in loss of consciousness, restricted activity, job transfer, absence from work, medical treatment beyond immediate first aid, or work injury or illness diagnosed by licensed healthcare provider:

- Form 300 (Log of Work-Related Injuries and Illnesses): Includes identification of the person with case number, employee's name, and title, and a description of the case with date of injury/illness onset, where the event occurred and description of the injury or illness including body part affected, and object/substance that caused injury or illness.
- Form 300A (Summary of Work-Related Injuries and Illnesses): Must be filed annually between February 1 and April 30 of the year following the year covered by the form. Includes a summary of number of cases, number of days away from work or on restricted work or transfer, and types of injuries and illnesses.
- Form 301 (Injury and Incident Report): Includes specific information about the injury, including information about the employee and healthcare provider, the type of injury, and the treatment. Must include a complete description of how the injury/illness occurred and the extent of the injury/illness.

Needlestick Safety and Prevention Act

OSHA's bloodborne pathogens standards comply with the **Needlestick Safety and Prevention Act (2000).** Employees must have an active voice in reviewing and selecting needle safety devices in order to reduce risk of injury, and a list of employee participants in the selection process must be on file. Each institution must maintain a needlestick and injury log that includes the following information:

- Description of how the incident occurred and the extent of injury.
- The brand and type of product involved in the incident.
- The location where the incident occurred.

All incidents involving needles and sharps must be reported and documented even if no serious injury or illness occurred as a result on the incident. All employees with possible exposure to bloodborne pathogens should receive hepatitis B vaccination.

SDS

Safety Data Sheets (SDS), formerly known as Material Safety Data Sheets (MSDS), explain how to handle caustic substances in the event of an accident or injury and provide pertinent information on the composition and toxic effects of the chemicals in the lab. SDS outline proper storage of chemicals, procedures for clean up, and dumping of caustic substances as well as procedures in the event of a chemical spill or injury and proper locations in the facility for clean-up. The SDS should also contain information indicating which substances may cause allergic effects or asthma from contact or inhalation. Emergency rescue services generally have SDS for common chemicals and products. Manufacturers and suppliers should have SDS on file and can be contacted for copies. OSHA/EPA Occupational Chemical Database provides links for SDS for some products. SDS are available from various other sources, including Toxicology Data Network (TOXNET), Pathogen Safety Data Sheets (biological hazards), and Poison Control centers.

Planning and Responding to Internal and External Disasters

Disaster planning should include plans for both internal and external disasters. Five critical elements of preparation include:

- Communication plans: includes phone trees or other notification systems and external notification of community agencies/resources.
- Essential supplies: IVs, dressing supplies, essential medications should be stockpiled.
- Staff roles and responsibilities: Staff members should be trained in disaster preparedness and understand their roles and responsibilities.
- Power/Utilities: Backup systems should provide power for up to 96 hours.
- Clinical patient care: Plans for provision of care under varying circumstances, including alternate plans.

Internal disasters, such as fires, flooding, storm damage, and terrorist attacks, often result in the evacuation of patients and the need for transportation services to transfer patients while external disasters, such as hurricanes, tornadoes, terrorist attacks, floods, pandemics, and transportation disasters, more often result in a large influx of patients and the need to discharge non-critical patients to make room for new patients, depending on the type of practice.

Active Shooters and Terrorist Bomb Attacks

With **active shooters,** standard protocol has been for emergency response services to wait until the police have removed the threat and secured the area before moving in to care for victims, leaving victims essentially on their own; however, this delay in treatment may result in death, so some authorities are now recommending that emergency response personnel enter the scene with police while wearing appropriate protective equipment although this does pose some risk, especially with additional shooters or secondary attack. With **terrorist bombing** and improvised explosive devices (IEDs), situational awareness is critical because multiple explosive devices (some undetonated) may be at the scene. IEDs may be inside backpacks, suitcases, and packages left unattended, but in emergency situations, other people often drop backpacks and packages and run. Additionally, people wearing suicide vests or belts may mix in with other victims or people escaping the blast area.

Path of Least Resistance

The **path of least resistance** is an important concept to understand for rescues, especially if they involve fire and any products of combustion (smoke, heat, gas). Fire's path of least resistance is usually vertical and upward although fire also spreads horizontally, especially if a vertical path is not available. It's for this reason that if there is a fire on the top floor of a building, the roof is breached to prevent horizontal spread. External factors, such as gusts of wind, can affect the path of least resistance. Water, on the other hand, also flows vertically, but downward and then horizontally if the downward flow is blocked. If rescuing patients from a building, they will often be found near the path of least resistance, such as a near a door or window. Patients should also be evacuated according to the path of least resistance; that is, the route that is the easiest and safest.

Decreasing Risks of Slips, Trips, and Falls

The CMAA should take an active role in creating a **safe workplace environment** and preventing accidents:

- <u>Slips</u>: Most slips occur when the floor is wet or lacks adequate traction. Common causes include spills (water, urine, soap), oily substances (leaking oil), loose rugs and mats, and excessive floor waxing. Slips are especially a risk during wet weather as people may track water or snow in from outside. Floors should be checked and kept clean and dry,
- <u>Trips</u>: Most trips occur when the foot encounters obstacles (wrinkled rugs, cables, cords, clutter), view/walkway is obstructed, or lighting is poor. Traffic areas should be kept clear of clutter and lighting checked. Uneven steps should have warning signs.
- <u>Falls</u>: Many falls result from slipping or tripping, but some occur from a height, such as a from a ladder or stairs. Patients who are unstable should always be assisted when walking and assisted at an appropriate pace.

Body Mechanics/Ergonomics

<u>Things to Avoid</u>
Proper body mechanics/**ergonomics** and prevention of repetitive strain injury include:

- Avoid bending at the waist to lift or reach for items. Stoop down with the knees bent.
- Avoid stretching overhead to reach for items on high shelves or out of reach (more than 20 inches). Use a step stool or grip tool with extension.
- Avoid pulling—push, roll, or slide instead.
- Avoid lifting—pull, push, roll, or slide instead.
- Avoid reaching, bending, or twisting to lift.
- Avoid lifting. Use lift devices rather than manually lifting heavy items and patients or get help.
- Avoid prolonged periods of repetitive activity, such as keyboarding or stocking materials and take note of numbness and tingling or discomfort (warning signs). Take frequent short breaks.

<u>Guidelines</u>

Ergonomics is the study of how to design work and products according to principles of body mechanics to avoid injury, especially in the workplace:

- Lift with leg muscles, not back.
- Hold weight close to body rather than at arm's length. Use the whole body to relieve strain on the arms and back.
- Flex at hips and knees, not waist.
- Maintain a straight back and avoid twisting.
- Assess weight and recognize limitations in lifting/carrying.
- Get help when necessary and communicate every step with partner ("Lift on the count of three").
- Maintain firm base of support with feet apart (shoulder width) to stabilize stance.
- Maintain line of gravity (imaginary line between center of gravity and ground) within the base of support.
- Stand close to the person or item to be lifted, bend knees and hips, and use the muscles in the legs to support weight rather than the back or arms.

Hazardous Materials

Hazardous materials are any that may cause harm (health or physical hazard) to humans or animals by themselves or through interaction with something else. Hazardous materials may be:

- <u>Chemical</u>: Include blister agents, blood agents, choking agents, nerve agents, asphyxiants, and irritants. These can enter the body through inhalation, absorption, ingestion, and injection.
- <u>Radiological</u>: Nuclear material, radioactive substances (alpha/beta particles).
- <u>Physical/Biological</u>: Infectious wastes, blood and other body fluids, biotoxins.

Almost any material or substance can be classified as hazardous depending on various factors, such as location, amount, and interactions. <u>Exposure</u> occurs when a person/animal comes in contact with the hazardous material and <u>contamination</u> is the residue resulting from exposure. <u>Absorption</u> is the method by which hazardous material enters the bloodstream. Exposure and contamination may result in immediate (blistering, itching, pain) or delayed responses (nausea, vomiting, cancer, lung disease).

Hazardous Waste

Hazardous waste is waste that poses a threat to the health of individuals or to the environment. OSHA provides definitions of and rules concerning handling of hazardous wastes. Hazardous wastes are classified according to characteristics:

- <u>Ignitable</u>: Liquids and non-liquids that can ignite and cause fires.
- <u>Corrosive</u>: Based on pH or the ability to corrode steel.
- <u>Reactive</u>: Wastes that are unstable, may react with water, or result in toxic gases. They may also explode.
- <u>Toxic</u>: Wastes that are harmful if ingested or absorbed.

Wastes may also be classified as listed wastes. These include wastes from manufacturing and industrial processes. Hazardous wastes are often produced in manufacturing, nuclear power plants (nuclear wastes), and healthcare facilities (needles, materials contaminated with body fluids).

Nuclear wastes are classified as mixed waste because they contain a radioactive component as well as a hazardous component. Hazardous wastes can result in disease (such as from needle punctures), injury (from fire and explosions), and death (from toxic exposure, disease).

Reporting Medicare/Medicaid Fraud

Medicare/Medicaid fraud may involve (1) billing for services not actually provided, (2) billing for patients not actually seen, (3) billing for unnecessary services, procedures, and tests, and (4) and upcoding (billing for a service at a higher level than that provided, such as billing for a complete physical exam when only a partial examination was carried out. According to CMS, about 10% of bills involve some type of fraud. Note that the whistleblower is protected by law and may be eligible for a reward. Procedures for reporting include:

- Medicare: Telephone report at 1-800-633-4227, TTY at 1-877-486-2048, online at the Office of the Inspector General or call directly at 1-800-447-8477 or TTY at 1-800-377-4950 or fax (up to 10 pages) to 1-800-223-8164 or Email (up to 10 pages) to HHSTips@oig.hhs.gov.
- Medicaid: Reports can be made by calling the Department of Social Services or the State Medicaid Agency in the state where the fraud occurred. Other options include the Medicaid Fraud hotline at 1-888-742-7248 or online at https://www.medicaidfraudhotline.com/.

Convictions may result in fines, prison terms, and/or loss of license to practice.

Insurance Models

Medicaid

Medicaid is a combined federal and state welfare program authorized by Title XIX of the Social Security Act to assist people with low income with payment for medical care. This program provides assistance for all ages, including children. Older adults receiving SSI are eligible as are others who meet state eligibility requirements. The Medicaid programs are administered by the individual states, which establish eligibility and reimbursement guidelines, so benefits vary considerably from one state to another. Older adults with Medicare are eligible for Medicaid as a secondary insurance. Expenses that are covered include inpatient and outpatient hospital services, physician payments, nursing home care, home health care, and laboratory and radiation services. Adults who are legal resident aliens are ineligible for Medicaid for 5 years after attaining legal resident status. Some states pay for preventive services, such as home and community-based programs aimed at reducing the need for hospitalization.

Medicare

Medicare, a federal health insurance program for those who have Social Security or bought into Medicare, provides payment to private healthcare providers, such as physicians and hospitals, but limits reimbursement. Physicians receive 80% of usual customary and reasonable (UCR) fees if they accept Medicare assignment. If they do not, they can charge up to 115% of what Medicare allows. Patients are responsible for the remaining 20% or up to 115% if the physicians do not accept Medicare. Parts include:

- Medicare A: Hospital insurance covers acute hospital, limited nursing home care and/or home health care as well as hospice care for the terminally ill. There is no premium for this part.
- Medicare B: Medical insurance covers physicians, advance practice nurses, laboratory, physical and occupational therapy. Patients must pay an annual deductible as well as monthly payments.

- <u>Medicare D</u>: Prescription drug plan covers part of the costs of prescription drugs at participating pharmacies. It is administered by private insurance companies, so monthly costs and benefits vary somewhat.

<u>Medicare Managed Care</u>

Medicare Managed Care is provided by a health maintenance organization (HMO), which receives payment for services rather than the traditional pay-for-service Medicare payment system. The Medicare HMO programs are available in only some areas and may vary in the type of services they provide. Typically, a person must choose or is assigned a primary care physician who serves as the gatekeeper to determine what other services or physicians the patient needs, and the patient must stay within the HMO network. To enroll, generally the person must be eligible for Medicare and not in end-stage renal disease or receiving hospice care. There is an open enrollment period each year during which a patient must apply for enrollment. Many HMOs have stopped accepting Medicare patients because the costs for care were so high, so many older adults do not have access to this type of program. Some programs have been successful in lowering costs by instituting preventive health programs.

<u>Medicare Preferred Providers and Other Plans</u>

Medicare has made a number of modifications to allow Medicare patients to access different types of programs in addition to typical pay-for-service care and managed care through HMOs:

- <u>Prospective payment system</u> (PPS) pays a set amount for patient care, depending upon diagnosis (diagnosis-related group or DRG).
- <u>Preferred provider organization</u> (PPO) provide discounted rates for those on Medicare who choose healthcare providers from a list of those who have agreed to accept Medicare assignment.
- <u>Private insurance pay-for-service Medicare plans</u> are contracted by Medicare and may provide more benefits, but the patient may be required to work individually with the insurance company to determine benefits and may be assessed an additionally monthly fee.
- <u>Specialty plans</u> are being developed in different areas, some focusing on increased preventive care.

<u>Tricare</u>

Tricare is the health care program serving active military, retired military, and their spouses and dependents. Tricare provides a number of different plans, depending upon location and eligibility. For those with Medicare, Tricare becomes the secondary insurer. If patients choose to opt out of Medicare (such as those with no insurance or private insurance), Tricare pays the amount equivalent to a secondary insurer (20% of allowable), and the patient is responsible for the rest. By law, all other insurances must pay before Tricare. Patients may access care at military treatment facilities (MTF) on space-available basis, but must enroll in Tricare Plus to receive primary care at MTFs. Those eligible for both Tricare and Veterans Affairs (VA) programs, may receive care at VA medical facilities if the service is covered under Tricare and the facility is part of the Tricare network, but the VA cannot bill Medicare, so costs not covered by Tricare must be paid by the patient even if the patient has Medicare coverage.

<u>Workers' Compensation</u>

The primary focus of **Workers' Compensation**, a type of insurance, is to return people to work as quickly and safely as possible. Worker's Compensation is intended for those who are injured on the job or whose health is impaired because of their jobs. Worker's Compensation provides 3 different types of benefits: cash to replace lost wages, reimbursement for medical costs associated with the injury, and death benefits to survivors. Worker's Compensation laws may vary somewhat from one state to another. In some states, the insurance carrier or the employer has the right to choose the healthcare provider, so knowledge of state laws is important. Separate records (medical and financial) must be maintained for patients covered under Worker's Compensation because requests for records related to the injury/illness only apply to records of the injury/illness. No other health information may be provided.

Health Insurance Claim Form

The Health Insurance Association of America has created a standardized health insurance claim form (**HCFA-1500**), which is usually acceptable to most insurance companies and similar to insurance companies own forms. HCFA-1500 is also the required form for Medicare claims, referred to as **CMS-1500**. Some insurance companies, however, insist on their own form. HCFA/CMS-1500 can be completed online and submitted electronically. HCFA/CMS 1500 has four sections:

- Patient: Demographic information, signature for release of medical records (authorization), and information related to whether the healthcare provider accepts assignment of benefits.
- Subscriber: Information about the holder of the insurance policy and relationship to the patient as well as information about the insurance coverage for employer-sponsored plans, including policy and patient ID numbers.
- Carrier: Information about primary and secondary insurance.
- Provider: Information about the services provided linked to the ICD-10-CM diagnostic codes for up to 4 diagnoses.

Health Insurance Billing Form

UB-04/CMS 1450 is the uniform billing form developed by CMS but now the standardized form used across the insurance industry for medical and mental health billing. The form is printed in red on white paper and is also available in an electronic form. Information from the patient's insurance card should be entered exactly as written. UB-04/CMS 1450 has 81 fields (form locators) that must be filled in, including information about the provider, the types of bill, the Federal tax umber of the organization, dates, demographic information about the patient, admission date and time, type of visit, source of admission, discharge time, discharge status, condition codes, accident state (if appropriate), responsible party information, value codes, revenue codes and description, HCPCS and HIPPS codes, service dates, service units, total charges, non-covered charges, information about the payer, health plan, and insured, employer information, diagnostic codes, PPS codes, POA indicator, and provider information.

Patient Education

Patients' Rights

Patients' and residents' Bill of Rights in relation to what they should expect from a healthcare organization are outlined in both standards of the Joint Commission and National Committee for Quality Assurance. Rights include:

- Respect for patient, including personal dignity and psychosocial, spiritual, and cultural considerations.
- Response to needs related to access and pain control.
- Ability to make decisions about care, including informed consent, advance directives, and end of life care.
- Procedure for registering complaints or grievances.
- Protection of confidentiality and privacy.
- Freedom from abuse or neglect.
- Protection during research and information related to ethical issues of research.
- Appraisal of outcomes, including unexpected outcomes.
- Information about organization, services, and practitioners.
- Appeal procedures for decisions regarding benefits and quality of care.
- Organizational code of ethical behavior.
- Procedures for donating and procuring organs/tissue.

Patient Self-Determination Act

According to the **Patient Self-Determination Act** (1990), competent patients have the right to refusal of care, and parents have the right to make this decision for minor children. If a patient refuses care, the healthcare provider should try to persuade the patient to agree to care by giving the reasons and possible consequences of refusal. The patient should be asked to sign the refusal form and a family member, police officer, or bystander should sign as a witness to the patient's signing or witness the refusal to sign. The healthcare provider should complete documentation of any assessment carried out and any refusal of the patient to assessment. The healthcare provider should carefully document the conversation between the healthcare provider and patient regarding refusal of care and consequences and should document the proposed care as well as the information the healthcare provider gave the patient about alternate care (such as visit to personal physician) and the willingness to return if the patient has a change of mind.

Communication Techniques to Assess Patient Understanding

Communication techniques used when assessing patient's understanding and communication include:

- Reflection: Refers to both the meaning of the patient's words and the emotions. If a patient states," I understand how to monitor my blood pressure," a reflecting question might be: "You feel confident that you know how to take your blood pressure and when to notify the physician?"
- Restatement: Restates or paraphrases something a patient said, "I've been having dizzy spells for two weeks?" Restatement might be: "You've been having dizzy spells for 2 weeks."

- Clarification: Asks for more information. If a patient states, "I haven't been feeling well," a clarifying question might be: "What exactly do you mean when you say you haven't been feeling well?"
- Feedback: Responds to something a patient has said or done, letting them know that the message/information was received: "You have kept very accurate records of your blood pressure and pulse."

Defense Mechanisms

Defense mechanisms are those coping methods that people use, often unconsciously, to relieve or prevent anxiety:

- Denial: Refusing to believe or recognize some painful truth or reality. Denial often involves failing to recognize the seriousness of disease (such as diabetes) or habits (such as smoking). Patients may seek other opinions or change doctors. Patients may see their own failings, opinions, actions in others and not recognizing them as personal. Projection often involves aggressive thoughts.
- Projection: Identifying personal impulses, unacceptable thoughts, and conflicting feelings in others. Patients may accuse healthcare providers of being rude to them when they are being rude.
- Rationalization: Attempting to justify or making excuses. Patients may try to find a rational/logical reason or cause for something even if there is none and may rationalize nonadherence to treatment.
- Repression: Unintentionally forgetting disturbing thoughts, feelings, or events. Patients may unconsciously fail to recall traumatic incidents/feelings. Feelings of guilt are often repressed.

Right to Refuse

The **right to refuse** services rests with adults, so ordinarily an adult (or an emancipated minor who has been granted the rights of adulthood) can refuse any medication, treatment, counseling, or placement although this is not always true. Court orders override these rights, and if the court has declared a person is incompetent, this person's guardian makes the decisions. Additionally, if the court has ordered specific treatment, therapy, or placement, then the patient must comply even against the patient's wishes. Children, including adolescents, have no rights to refusal, but they should be consulted as much as possible, and their wishes should be respected and incorporated into the plan of care. For example, if an adolescent does not want to have a particular treatment, then options should be explored because forcing an adolescent to do something often results in poor outcomes.

Patient's Rights and Responsibilities

People are empowered to act as their own advocates when they have a clear understanding of their **rights and responsibilities.** These should be given (in print form) and/or presented (audio/video) to parents/guardians on admission to healthcare or as soon as possible:

- Rights should include competent, non-discriminatory medical care that respects privacy and allows participation in decisions about care and the right to refuse care. They should have clear understandable explanations of treatments, options, and conditions, including outcomes. They should be apprised of transfers, changes in care plan, and advance directives. They should have access to medical records information about charges.

- Responsibilities should include providing honest and thorough information about health issues and medical history. Parents/guardians should ask for clarification if they don't understand information that is provided to them, and they should follow the plan of care that is outlined or explain why that is not possible.

Ownership of Medical Records

The **medical record,** whether electronic or paper, belongs to the patient's physician who was responsible for the making of the record and the facility or organization, such as a hospital where the record was made. However, the information contained within the medical record belongs to the patient under the rules of HIPAA. Therefore, patients have a right to look at the medical record and to review the information it contains and are entitled to a copy of the medical record but not the medical record itself, which must be stored by the physician or facility/organization. Holders of the patient's medical record have, according to HIPAA regulations, up to 30 days to comply with a request for records and can apply for an additional 30-day extension. Some state laws have a shorter timetable that applies, so the CMAA should review state requirements. For example, in California, patients must be able to review a record within 5 days and must receive a copy within 15 days of request.

ADA

The 1992 **Americans with Disabilities Act (ADA)** is civil rights legislation that provides the disabled, including those with mental impairment, access to employment and the community. The ADA prevents discrimination against employees or potential employees for organizations with =/>15 employees because of disabilities. These provisions are enforced by the Equal Employment Opportunity Commission (EEOC). Employers are only allowed to ask applicants if they need accommodations, not if they have disabilities, and individual accommodations must be made. Accommodations that may apply to a CMAA or others can include:

- Alterations in work station.
- Speech recognition software.
- Screen magnifying software.
- Optical character recognition systems.
- Video captioning.
- Braille readers and screen readers.
- Adapted keyboards and on-screen keyboard.
- TTYs (text telephones).
- Amplification systems.

People who are disabled are entitled to assistive technology that will allow them to function but are not entitled to jobs that they are unable to do even with assistive devices or accommodations. Most computer operating systems now incorporate assistive technology (such as screen readers).

Disability Accommodations in the Medical Office

According to **ADA regulations**, the medical office must ensure that the office is accessible by those with disabilities. Requirements include:

- Door handles must be accessible by those in a wheelchair.
- Ramps must be available so that disabled patients can enter and exit buildings.
- Doors and hallways must be adequate to allow entering, exiting, and maneuvering. Doors should be 32 inches wide and able to open to 90 degrees.

- Telephones, drinking fountains, and bathrooms must be wheelchair accessible.
- Multi-story buildings must have elevators.
- Disabled persons must be able to access and use all services that non-disabled persons can access and use in a building.
- Disabled patients should be examined on an accessible examining table (adjustable to height of 17 to 19 inches from the floor) and not in a wheelchair. A clear space of 30 by 48 inches should be next to the accessible examining table to allow wheelchair access. A 60 by 60 inches circular or T-shaped space should be available in the room so that the wheelchair can carry out a 180-degree turn.
- Healthcare providers cannot refuse to treat a patient with disabilities because of inconvenience.
- Staff should receive training in caring for and treating disabled patients.

Medication Legislation

Act/Agency	Purpose
Pure Food and Drug Act	Consumer protection act intended to prevent manufacture, sale, and transportation of adulterated foods, drugs, and alcoholic beverages.
Federal Food, Drug, and Cosmetic Act	Provides authority to the FDA to oversee food, drug, and cosmetic safety.
Harrison Narcotic Act	Provides authority for regulation and taxation of production, importation, and distribution of coca/opium products, such as narcotics.
Controlled Substances Act	Establishes US drug policy and 5 schedules under which drugs are classified, implemented by the Drug Enforcement Administration and Food and Drug Administration.
Food and Drug Administration	Consumer protection agency that protects public health through control and supervision of drugs, vaccines, blood transfusions, medical devices, cosmetics, foods, tobacco, and dietary supplements.
Drug Enforcement Agency	Law enforcement agency, part of Department of Justice, enforces the Controlled Substances Act and combats drug smuggling/use.

Informed Consent

Guidelines

Patients or family must provide **informed consent** for all treatment the patient receives. This includes a thorough explanation of all procedures and treatment and associated risks. Patients/family should be apprised of all options and allowed input on the type of treatments. Patients/family should be apprised of all reasonable risks and any complications that might be life threatening or increase morbidity. The American Medical Association has established guidelines for informed consent:

- Explanation of diagnosis.
- Nature and reason for treatment or procedure.
- Risks and benefits.
- Alternative options (regardless of cost or insurance coverage).
- Risks and benefits of alternative options.
- Risks and benefits of not having a treatment or procedure.
- Providing informed consent is a requirement of all states.

The requirement for informed consent may be waived in life-threatening situations and if the EMR cannot obtain informed consent because the patient cannot communicate and legal consent cannot be obtained.

<u>Conditions for Consent</u>

The **conditions for consent** for care and decision-making capacity include:

- 18 years or older: Those who are younger may have the right to give consent for all or some medical treatment in some states. Laws vary. For example, the age of consent for medical treatment in Alabama is 14.
- Mentally competent to make decisions: May be impaired by mental disability, injury, illness, or substance abuse (intoxication).
- Court emancipated minor.
- Military service.
- Marriage.

Consent may be expressed in written or verbal form if the patient is able to give informed consent or may be implied for both minors and adults, such as when provided care in an emergent situation in which the patient is unable to give consent. Parents or caregivers give consent for minors below the age of 18 unless they have been emancipated. If parents or caregivers are unavailable to give consent, life-saving emergent care, general medical assessment, and medical care to prevent further injury or harm can be provided without consent (*in loco parentis*).

<u>Obtaining Consent from Legal Guardian</u>

In some cases, a **legal guardian** must give consent for treatment and release of records rather than the patient. The three most common types of legal guardians are (1) those that are responsible for a person who is incapacitated, such as an elderly adult with dementia or a patient with severe mental illness; (2) those who are responsible for minors, such as the parents; and (3) those who are responsible for children and adults who are developmentally disabled, such as those with severe cognitive impairment. The guardians for adults should have court documents showing they have the right to make decisions for the patient, but parents of minor children are assumed by law to have this right. Once guardianship is verified, consent is obtained in the same manner as consent would be obtained from the patient. The guardian must have a complete understanding of the purpose of the consent and the implications.

Negligence, Abandonment, Assault, Battery, Kidnapping, and False Imprisonment

The four necessary elements of **negligence** (failure to follow standards of care) are:

- <u>Duty of care</u>: The defendant (healthcare provider) had a duty to provide adequate care and/or protect the plaintiff's (patient's) safety.
- <u>Breach of duty</u>: The defendant failed to carry out the duty to care, resulting in danger, injury, or harm to the plaintiff.
- <u>Damages</u>: The plaintiff experienced illness or injury as a result of the breach of duty.
- <u>Causation</u>: The plaintiff's illness or injury is directly caused by the defendant's negligent breach of duty.

Abandonment occurs if the paramedic withdraws from providing care contrary to patient's desire or knowledge and fails to arrange for appropriate care by others, resulting in harm to the patient. **Assault** occurs if a paramedic threatens a patient in some way that the patient becomes fearful of harm while **battery** occurs when the paramedic intentionally injures a patient, such as by hitting or

- 69 -

shoving the person. **Kidnapping** is forcefully transporting a patient and **false imprisonment** is preventing a patient from leaving.

Types of Negligence

Negligence indicates that *proper care* has not been provided, based on established standards. *Reasonable care* uses rationale for decision-making in relation to providing care. State regulations regarding negligence may vary but all have some statutes of limitation, governmental immunity, and Good Samaritan laws may provide defense. Types of negligence include:

- Negligent conduct: An individual failed to provide reasonable care or to protect/assist another, based on standards and expertise.
- Gross negligence: Willfully providing inadequate care while disregarding the safety and security of another.
- Contributory negligence: injured party contributing to his/her own harm.
- Comparative negligence: The percentage amount of negligence attributed to each individual involved.

If the charge of negligence is supported, the patient may collect physical (lost earnings due to injury), psychological (pain and suffering), and punitive damages.

Reporting Unsafe Activities and Behaviors in the Workplace

Each organization should have protocols in place for the reporting of **unsafe activities and behaviors**. In most cases, reports are made to the CMAA's immediate supervisor. Unsafe activities and behaviors include:

- Failure to follow standard procedures: Taking shortcuts to save time often increases risk to staff and patients.
- Lack of understanding/information: Carrying out tasks without completely understanding what is expected or needed can result in doing the task incorrectly. Overconfidence can lead to attempting activities for which the person is not adequately trained.
- Inadequate housekeeping: Improper cleaning can lead to risk of falls (from clutter) and infection (from improper disinfection).
- Noncompliance with safety protocols: Ignoring safety rules (oxygen storage, smoke alarms) can put everyone at risk.
- Distractions: Emotional upset, pain, and illness can all increase risk of errors.
- Inadequate planning: Last minute assignments, constantly changing assignments and duties, and inadequate preparation all can lead to unsafe behaviors.

Disclosure of Errors in Patient Care

Each healthcare facility/office should have established protocols for **disclosure of errors in patient care,** and the CMAA must always immediately report any error to a supervising nurse or physician so that steps can be taken to prevent further problems or injury to the patient involved. An incident report should be filled out to document the error, initiated by the person involved or closest to the patient when the incident occurred. The report should be detailed, listing the date, time, and exact sequence of events as well as any witnesses. The report should be reviewed by a supervisor. If the patient is aware of the error (such as when a CMAA accidentally strikes a patient), the CMAA should immediately apologize and ensure that the patient is examined by a nurse or

- 70 -

physician. For more serious errors or those for which the patient may be unaware, risk management may have protocols in place that preclude discussing the error for liability reasons.

Core Ethical Principles

Core ethical principles include:

- <u>Beneficence</u>: Performing actions that are for the purpose of benefitting another person. In the care of a patient, any procedure or treatment should be done with the ultimate goal of benefitting the patient.
- <u>Nonmaleficence</u>: Providing care in a manner that does not cause direct intentional harm to the patient. Care must be intended only for good effect, and good effects must have more benefit than bad effects that result.
- <u>Autonomy</u>: The right of the individual to make decisions about his/her own care. In the case of children, the child cannot make autonomous decisions, so the parents serve as the legal decision maker.
- <u>Justice</u>: Relates to the distribution of the limited resources of healthcare benefits to the members of society. Resources must be distributed fairly and decisions made according to what is most just.
- <u>Privacy/Confidentiality</u>: Protecting information (conversations, assessments) and body (close door, pull curtains, use drapes to avoid exposing patient) and protecting personal information about a patient and the patient's health condition.

Ethical Principles and Moral Obligations Involved in Providing Care

Ethics is a branch of philosophy that studies morality, concepts of right and wrong. Applied ethics is the use of ethical principles, such as autonomy (right to self-determination), beneficence (acting to benefit another), nonmaleficence (doing no harm), verity (being truthful), and justice (equally distributing resources/care). Ethical conflicts may occur because of differences in cultural and ethical values but may also result from decisions that must be made regarding care, such as whether to provide CPR in a wilderness situation when the treatment is likely futile, situations involving triage where some patients are given priority over others, situations that involve professional misconduct (such as healthcare personnel being abusive toward patients), and incidents of patient dumping because the patient has inadequate insurance or ability to pay. Healthcare personnel have a moral obligation to make decisions about care in good faith and in the patients' best interest.

Medical Assisting Code of Ethics and Code of Conduct

The American Association of Medical Assistants (AAMA) published the **Medical Assisting Code of Ethics** to guide practice for those working as medical assistants. The Code requires that medical assistants pledge to:

- Provide service to patients that shows respect.
- Maintain confidentiality and divulge information only within the parameters of the law.
- Uphold the principles of the profession.
- Participate in activities to promote community health and well-being.

Additionally, medical assistants are expected to adhere to a **Code of Conduct**, which requires that they:

- Carry out duties with integrity and maintain high standards in both personal and professional conduct.
- Accept that they are responsible for their own actions.
- Carry out practice with fairness and honesty.
- Practice within the framework of the law and regulations.
- Encourage others in the field to maintain high standards and professional behavior.

Decision-Making Models

Do no harm	This model is based on nonmaleficence, the requirement that a treatment provided do no harm; however, by their nature, some treatments can and often do harm patients, so the underlying intent and goal of treatment must be considered when making decisions. For example, CPR may be carried out to save a patient's life, but even if done with correct technique, it may still result in rib fractures.
In good faith	The motive for a decision should be honest and fair and decisions made with sincere intention to do good even though the outcome may be negative. For example, healthcare personnel may provide a treatment for a patient in good faith although the treatment proves to be ineffective.
Patient's best interest	Making a decision in the patient's best interests includes considering the patient's or parents' (in the case of children) wishes, the best clinical judgment, the best choice of various options, the chances for improvement/decline, and religious/cultural preferences.

Financial Terminology

Copayments, Deductibles, and Coinsurance

Copayments are fixed costs that the patient must pay for health care services (such as doctor's office visits or physical therapy treatments) after the patient has paid any required **deductible**, which is a fixed amount that the patient is responsible for before the insurance company begins to cover the costs of healthcare. Both deductibles and copayments may vary, depending on the type of insurance plan the patient has. Copayment costs are usually indicated on the patient's insurance card. With **co-insurance**, instead of a fixed copayment, the insured pays a percentage of medical costs. For example, the insurance company may cover 80% and the individual 20%. Each patient should be asked about their copayments, co-insurance, and deductibles so that money can be collected. Each practice should have a policy outlining steps to take if a patient cannot pay a copayment or deductible at the time of the visit. For example, arrangements may be made for the patient to make payments or to pay at a later time. Most practices accept credit cards as well.

Allowed Amount

Allowed amount (AKA allowable charge) is the dollar amount that an insurance company is willing to pay for a specific service. For example, the insurance company may be willing to pay only $50 for a test. If a healthcare provider charges more than this amount, the patient may be responsible for the balance if the provider has not agreed to accept the amount as payment in full. Additionally, if a patient wants to visit a physician that is outside of the patient's approved network of physicians, the patient may receive large bills. Therefore, it's essential that patients understand the allowed amounts of their insurance policies and always verify that healthcare providers are in their approved network of providers. The CMAA should advise new patients if a healthcare provider they wish to see is outside of their network or a specialist is outside of their network.

Insurance Models

Types and Characteristics of Health Insurance	
HMO	With health maintenance organizations (HMOs), a primary care provider (PCP) coordinates care and referrals to a network of healthcare providers. The individual has little choice and requires a referral from the PCP to see a specialist. Plans may provide preventive care but may also require co-payments and deductible.
PPO	With a preferred provider organization (PPO) an individual can choose to see any healthcare provider, including specialists, in a network of healthcare providers. The individual is not usually required to select a PCP but may have to pay co-payments and deductible, depending on the plan. Individuals can usually see healthcare providers outside of the network but reimbursement is typically lower, so the individual may have to pay part of costs.
EPO	The exclusive provider organization (EPO) is similar to PPO in that the individual can see any physician within a network except that the individual does not have the option of seeing a healthcare provider outside of the network except in emergency situations.
POS	Point of service plans (POSs) are combined HMOs and PPOs. The individual has a PCP within a network, and the PCP makes referrals, but the individual can see out-of-network healthcare providers; however, the individual must pay part of cost for out-of-network providers.
HDHP	High deductible health plans (HDHPs) may be HMOs, PPOs, or EPOs but are characterized by a high deductible before the insurance begins to reimburse for care. People with low income often select option to avoid catastrophic costs but may end up with large bills for healthcare services.

Methods to Maximize Reimbursement

Methods to maximize reimbursement include:

- Timely recording of information and sending of claims.
- Utilizing care managers to determine the most cost-effective care plan.
- Utilizing standardized billing codes (CPT, ICD).
- Ensuring that the healthcare provider's National Provider Identifier (NPI) is present on all claims.
- Updating systems promptly when new coding (such as ICD-10) and billing regulations (such as pay-for-performance) are issued rather than waiting for the end of the grace period so that problems can be identified and corrected early.
- Ensuring that the present on admission (POA) Medicare severity diagnosis related group (MS-DRG) diagnosis is correct to avoid a different discharge diagnosis.
- Monitoring quality of care to prevent complications and reduce costs related to the Do Not Pay List.
- Sending claims in the correct form and to the correct address for different entities: insurance companies, Medicaid, Medicare.

- 73 -

ABN

An **Advance Beneficiary Notice of Noncoverage** (ABN) (Form CMS-R-131) is given to Original Medicare and Medicare Fee-for-Service patients (<u>not</u> Medicare Managed care or Private Fee-for-Service patients) by healthcare providers is to notify them that an item or service is not covered by Medicare (usually meaning that supplementary insurance will also not cover the item or service). ABNs may also be issued if the patient wants a service or item that is not deemed medically necessary at that time but is a service or item that is generally covered by Medicare. ABNs are not required to inform patients of services that are never covered by Medicare, such as acupuncture. For those on Medicare Advantage Plans, CMS does not require that the patient be provided an ABN for noncovered items or service, but the healthcare provider may do so as a courtesy to alert patients. When ABNs are provided on a voluntary basis to notify patients of noncovered items/services, the patients should not sign the form or indicate a choice of options.

EOB

The **Explanation of Benefits** (EOB) is a report sent by the insurance company to the patient that describes payments made, reduced, or denied as well as deductibles paid and allowed amounts and patient's responsibilities. The amount billed may be the standard fee, while the allowed amount may represent that agreed to by the healthcare provider, so the patient is not required to pay the difference unless the insurance company and the healthcare provider have not agreed to assignment of benefits. If there is coordination of benefits (COB), such as when there is another insurance such as Medicare, the EOB should indicate this. In this example, a patient with Medicare as primary insurance and Model Insurance as a secondary insurance had an X-ray that was billed for $54.00 but the fee was adjusted to $11.28 because of assignment of benefits. Medicare, under coordination of benefits paid $8.99 and the insurance company paid $2.29.

Model Insurance Explanation of Benefits Service period 02/05/19 through 02/05/19							
Date	Service	Billed Amt.	Allowed Amt.	Deduct.	Copay	Plan paymt.	Patient respon.
02-05-19	Radiology	$54.00	$11.28	$0.00	$0.00	$2.29	$0.00
Totals: COB $8.99		$54.00	$11.28	$0.00	$0.00	$2.29	
Paid amount:						$2.29	

Documentation

Documentation must always be done during patient care or immediately afterward to ensure that no important information is forgotten or overlooked. The certified CMAA should make objective observations as opposed to subjective:

- Subjective: "Patient in severe pain from right arm injury."
- Objective: "Patient moaning and holding right arm."

All encounters (in-person, telephone, email) must be documented. Patient's acceptance of treatment should be documented, explaining the treatment and the patient response. Compliance or lack of compliance with the treatment regimen must be documented at each visit and contact. When appropriate, a consent form must be signed and witnessed and entered into the permanent record. If a patient refuses treatment or refuses to follow through with advice, this information must be documented along with the patient's reason and the patient asked to sign the statement as well if utilizing a paper record. In some cases, the patient may be asked to sign a "Refusal of Medical Advice" document, which is stored in the permanent record.

Preparation for Office Opening

Preparations for **office opening** usually begin at the end of the preceding workday when the daily appointment schedule for the next day is filled out or printed and the charts (if paper) are pulled and organized. If laboratory reports, imaging, or consultations had been ordered prior to the scheduled patient visit, the medical record should be checked to make sure that the appropriate reports have been received and are in the medical record for the healthcare provider to review. For patients scheduled for procedures that require medications, supplies, or equipment, these should be assembled and readied for use as much as possible. On opening, the doors should be unlocked, lights turned on, ventilation (air conditioning, heating) checked, equipment (such as computers) turned on, petty cash counted, and the waiting area straightened and ready. Floors should be checked to make sure there is no clutter and a tissue supply placed in the waiting area. Telephone, email, and faxes should be checked for messages and answering services contacted.

General Office Policies and Procedures

Checking and Forwarding Internal and External Messages

As soon as possible after opening the office, the **messages** received per telephone, email, text message, and fax should be checked, noting the time the message was received. Any emergency messages, such as a message left from a patient complaining of severe abdominal pain or bleeding, should be attended to first. Messages may be forwarded to the appropriate person (such as the physician, nurse practitioner, or billing person) either electronically or on paper message forms. Any urgent messages should be pointed out verbally in person or by phone to the person to whom the message is directed so the message is not overlooked or the response delayed. The person receiving the message should document the response.

Message		
To: Dr. Jones		
Date: 2-8	Time:	7:30 AM
From: Jasper Wood		
Telephone #: 201-6882		
Message: BP has been ranging from		
136/88 to 124/82 and pulse 68-72 with		
new medication.		
URGENT _____	Called	X
Returned call _____		
Response: TC to pt. 8:30 AM.		
Continue med. Noted in med. record.		

Cleaning the Reception Area

The **reception area** is usually the first place a patient enters, so it should always be kept neat, clean, uncluttered, and inviting. Housekeeping staff is generally responsible for heavy duty cleaning, such as scrubbing the floors or vacuuming and dusting, but the reception area can become very messy during office hours as people waiting scatter magazines and leave cups, trash, and water bottles about the area. The area should have adequate individual seating for peak hours and adequate lighting. The reception area should be checked and straightened on a regular basis, such as every 2 hours, or when it's obviously in disarray. Magazines should be up-to-date and of general interest to the public and tattered and torn magazines discarded. Practices that often include children should have books, puzzles, and/or toys available to keep children occupied, but these must be routinely sanitized to avoid the spread of infection.

Backing up Data

Data should be encrypted, backed up, and transferred to an offsite data storage area at least weekly. Hardware systems that are essential, including servers, routers, and Internet connections, should be duplicated. All backup systems should be tested regularly, at least on a monthly basis. Because hardware and software are likely to fail at some point, redundant systems are critical. Backup is necessary to ensure that information is not lost in the event of a system breakdown or failure. If data become corrupted, the organization should have a policy in place to revert to backup, accessing data that was stored prior to the data becoming corrupted as this will result in minimal need for re-entry of data. Data must always be assessed and protected during any types of system changes, such as migration of data to another system, updates, new applications, new types of storage devices, or changes in coding systems.

Ordering Supplies

Inventory

Inventory is stock of materials or equipment on hand. Inventories should be done at least once a year or more often. In many cases, reordering is done when inventory of a particular item drops to a certain pre-established count. Just-in-time ordering, however, waits until inventory stock is almost depleted. These types of automatic reordering of supplies are easier with computerized inventories. In some cases, practices have open accounts that can be used for small purchases without bidding. For larger purchases (especially in public institutions), a responsible person should state exactly (including brand names when appropriate) those items to be purchased on a bid form. Then, the bids are sent to prospective bidders (at least 3) in a competitive bid process. Organizations vary in what bids are acceptable. Some only accept the low bid, others the best bid (such as those supplying brand names rather than substituting with generic). Many organizations have private purchase plans that allow them to purchase directly without bids or to lease equipment, which is less expensive initially.

Inventory terms include:

- FIFO (first in, first out): Inventory is placed so that the oldest items are used first, especially important for items that are dated or perishable. This is the opposite of LIFO (last in, first out), which is used primarily for perishable items with a very limited shelf life.
- Trigger level: AKA the reorder level (level at which replenishments must be ordered).
- PAR (periodic automatic replenishment): The safety stock level, the minimum level to which the inventory can fall and still meet supply needs.
- Standing order: Replenishments are provided on a regularly scheduled basis, such as every 2 weeks. Standard orders include the frequency and the quantity although this can be adjusted if necessary.
- Expiration: Date by which an item is no longer usable, such as the expiration date on vacutainers.

Backorders and Rotation

Supply and inventory control aim to have adequate supplies on hand but to avoid oversupplies with a goal of 8 to 12 inventory turns per year with shelf lives no longer than 3 months for expendable (consumable) supplies. For that reason, expiration dates must be considered when managing inventory because outdated supplies, including medications, must be disposed of. New supplies should be placed behind those already stocked so that the supplies are rotated according to expiration date. Backorders can pose a problem if orders are placed at the last minute, resulting in the need to order from different suppliers or to substitute other supplies. A record of backorders should be maintained to determine if there are patterns in the types of backorders and the timing of backorders. Critical supplies should be maintained at a higher inventory level than those used less frequently. All shipments received should be checked for completeness and inspected for damage. The projected life expectancy of nonexpendable supplies (equipment) should be factored into purchases.

Greeting Patients Upon Arrival

Patients should be immediately acknowledged upon **arrival**, even if only briefly. If unable to attend to the person, the CMAA should greet the person ("Good morning") and indicate the need for a wait ("Please have a seat, and I'll be with you shortly"). Then, ask the patient's name and appointment time and verify if the patient is a new or returning patient and then check the patient's name against the appointment schedule to ensure the patient has the correct date and time. If the patient's name does not appear on the schedule, the CMAA should check records to determine the correct date and time and advise the patient. If time is available in the schedule, the patient may be added to the day's schedule and the previous appointment canceled to avoid the patient's having to make another trip. If the patient's actual appointment time was missed, the patient should be so advised and informed of any no-show charge.

Telephone Equipment/Functions

Telephone equipment/functions include:

- Speakerphone: Using handsfree communication allows the CMAA to carry out other duties, such as entering data into a computer, while speaking, but it also allows others to listen in, and the information may be covered by HIPAA regulations, especially if speaking with a patient. The caller should always be advised when a speakerphone is to be used and who else is present and can hear the exchange.
- Voice mail: Patients often dislike leaving voice messages and may leave incomplete messages, such as forgetting to give their name or telephone number. Voice mail instructions should be concise and clearly state needed information: Name, telephone number, and reason for calling. Voice mails should be answered as soon as possible.
- Call forwarding: When transferring a call to another person, the caller should be advised: "I'm going to transfer your call to Dr. Smith."
- Call hold: Placing a call on hold allows the CMAA to answer another call or to find information, but the caller should be advised that the call will be put on hold and for the estimated period of time as call hold is often frustrating for people, who may simply hang up and call back.

Telephone Calls Often Received by a Practice/Organization

Telephone calls often received by a practice/organization include:

- Requests for directions: Directions should be printed so they can be easily read over the telephone. If directions and/or a map are available online, the CMAA may over to send a text message or email with a link.
- Questions about bills: The CMAA should ask the nature of the question to determine whether the call needs to be forwarded to another person or can be answered directly. If information must be accessed, the caller may be placed on hold briefly. If billing is done by an outside agency, the CMAA should provide contact information for that agency. Before giving information, the CMAA should ask for identifying information, such as the caller's name, address, and date of birth.
- Questions about fees: Some callers want to know costs before making or keeping an appointment, so the CMAA should have a list of fees near the telephone and should provide the information, but the CMAA should ask first if the caller has insurance as the fees may vary depending on the carrier.

- Questions regarding participation in insurance plans: Callers often want to know if a healthcare provider is a member of their preferred provider network, so the CMAA should keep this information near the telephone and should be knowledgeable about any networks to which the healthcare provider is a member.
- Requests for results of diagnostic procedures: Before giving results, the CMAA should check with the healthcare provider to verify that results can be given to the patient or whether the healthcare provider needs to respond to the patient by phone or appointment. The CMAA should not give the patient news that may be devastating, such as news that cancer has recurred, as this is the responsibility of the healthcare provider. Before giving any results, the CMAA must verify the identity of the caller to ensure there is no HIPAA violation.
- Questions about insurance coverage/billing: Callers often call with questions about insurance, such as how and when they pay charges, so the CMAA should be knowledgeable about basic insurance procedures and the patient's right to appeal denials.
- Reports of condition/changes: Patients may call to report a new condition, a change in condition, or a progress report, such as current blood pressure. The CMAA should assure the patient that the information will be provided to the healthcare provider, and the information should be entered into the patient's medical record. If the report is negative and of concern (increased bleeding, pain), then the healthcare provider should be informed immediately and the patient placed on hold while the CMAA reports and gets instructions for the patient, or the CMAA should verify the patient's telephone number and advise the patient to expect a return call.
- Questions about referrals: Both patients and other healthcare providers may call requesting referrals. For example, a patient may want a referral to a specialist, such as a dermatologist. Some provider networks require that the primary care physician serve as gatekeeper and authorize all referrals. If the patient has not been recently seen, the patient may need to make an appointment before receiving a referral. Other healthcare providers may call to ask advice about referrals or may have been contacted by a patient who first needs a referral. If the healthcare provider has prepared a list of preferred referrals, the CMAA may refer to that list, but the healthcare provider should always be advised if information about referrals is given out. If a patient requests a referral or if a referral is given to a patient, this information should always be entered in the patient's medical record.
- Complaints: A patient or family member may call with complaints about services or bills, and the CMAA must avoid responding defensively or arguing. In some cases, the caller may be confused about a statement or other issue, and simply explaining or clarifying may defuse the situation. The best approach is to assure the caller of a willingness to help, "Let me see what I can do to help you/answer your questions." If the caller becomes abusive or threatening, then the CMAA should ask the caller to wait and refer the call to the healthcare provider or office manager.
- Requests for release of information: Before giving out any information, the CMAA must verify that the patient has signed a release of information form that allows the caller access and should verify that the type of information and the dates involved are covered by the release form.

Managing Emergency Situations Via Telephone

Some states have very specific guidelines as to which healthcare professional are able to **screen patients by telephone** or to give directions, so the CMAA must be aware of state guidelines. CMAAs, who are not trained or licensed to diagnose or give medical advice, can generally screen telephone calls but must be knowledgeable about the types of questions to ask and should follow a screening manual when taking calls to ensure consistency. The screening manual should list the

- 79 -

appropriate questions to ask depending on the patient's complaints/issues and indicate which responses require intervention of other healthcare providers, such as RN or emergency medical personnel (9-1-1). When using a screening manual, the CMAA should not deviate from the manual and should immediately consult a nurse or physician if the patient's complaints are not in the manual or the CMAA has concerns (such as the inability to make an immediate appointment for a patient in distress).

Correspondence

Basic Block Form Letter

The **block format** for letters is the most commonly used format for business letters although some may modify the format slightly, such as by placing the date on the opposite side. The parts of a letter include (1) a heading with the name and address and sometimes the telephone number and/or email address of the sender, (2) the date, (3) the recipient's name and address, (4) a salutation ("Dear Ms. Black," (4) body of the letter with the lines single-spaced and double-spaced between paragraphs, (5) closing ("Sincerely yours,"), (6) signature of sender printed with 4 lines left blank between the closing and the printed signature for the sender to sign, and (7) notation ("SJ:ma"). In some cases, a subject line (preceded by the word *Subject* or *Re* for "regarding") is placed between the salutation and the body of the letter ("Subject: Scheduled colonoscopy"). One-inch margins (right and left) are standard.

```
          Jones Medical Practice
              224 X Street
           San Jose, CA 94088

February 6, 2019

Ms. Susan Black
1180 Mountain Road
Silver City, CA  93999

Dear Ms. Black,


xxxxxxxxxxxxxxxxxxxxxxxxxxxxxxxxx
xxxxxxxxxxxxxxxxxxxxxxxxxxx.

xxxxxxxxxxxxxxxxxxxxxxxxxxxxxxxxx
xxxxxxxxx.

Sincerely yours,


Seth Jones, MD

SJ:ma
```

Types of Letters

A healthcare provider may send and receive many different **types of letters** and should have templates for each type to save time. The letters may be written (usually per word processing program on the computer) by the healthcare provider but may also be dictated and typed by a CMAA. Most letters are written in block format or modified block format without paragraph indentations. In some cases, the CMAA may be authorized to compose and send some types of letters, such as reminders of appointments or notification of missed appointments. Common letters in healthcare include:

- Consultation letters.
- Correspondence to patient, such as a letter to describe a pathology report after surgery.
- Billing letters.
- Letters regarding no-shows and missed appointments.
- Termination of services letters.
- Letters to insurance companies.

Before a letter is sent, it should always be spell-checked and grammar-checked and reviewed to ensure it contains no errors.

Business Tools

Templates

A **template** is a file that contains the basic structure of a specific type of document. For example, there are templates available in word processing programs for business letters, FAX cover sheets, and event calendars. Additionally, numerous templates are available for free online. Templates are available not only for documents but also for websites. People can design templates to meet specific needs, setting up the format, margins, font style, and font size. Once the template is set up, then no further formatting is required. Templates save time and simplify documentation. Templates are especially valuable if different individuals must produce the same type of document because the templates ensure that the individuals will use the same format. Templates make it easier to obtain needed information from a document and to combine information from various documents.

Email Systems

Email may be accessed in a number of ways:

- <u>Directly through a web browser</u>, such as Internet Explorer. Safari, Firefox, Edge, or Chrome. In this case, there is no storage of mail or backup on the person's computer because access is completely through the Internet. This type of access is generally free of charge.
- <u>Through an email client</u>, such as Microsoft Office Outlook. These systems provide backup and may offer more services, such as calendars and integration with other software. Outlook is part of MSN Office applications (which include MSN Word and Excel) and must be purchased, leased, or rented.
- <u>Through software applications</u>, such as Windows 8 Mail. This is similar to email through an email patient but is not part of a package of other applications.

Microsoft Office

Microsoft Office is a group of software applications that are sold together as a package. MSN Office is in common use in both home and businesses. The package includes:

- <u>Word</u>: Word processing program that allows one to produce a wide variety of documents. Templates available for various types of business communications, such as fax sheets and business letters.
- <u>Excel</u>: Spreadsheet that allows one to record data, make calculations, and present data in charts and graphs.
- <u>PowerPoint</u>: Slideshow presentation application that allows one to develop informational electronic slideshows that include pictures, videos, text, and audio.

- <u>Outlook</u>: Email handling service that integrates with other applications.
- <u>Access</u>: Database application that allows one to organize information.
- <u>Publisher</u>: Desk-top publishing application allows one to produce newsletters and other publications.

<u>Word Processing</u>

Word processing is using a computer software program to create or edit a document. Most word processing programs, such as MS Word and Google Docs, provide a variety of templates and include spell checkers and grammar checkers. Word processing programs can create and import a number of different types of files, indicated by the extension at the end of the file's name:

- .jpeg/.jpg (image): Used to compress files for photographs.
- .gif (image): Used to compress files for drawings and illustrations and illustrated animations.
- docx (xml document): Used for documents, generally those created by word processing programs.
- .txt: (text) Used for text files that can contain no special formatting.
- .rtf: (rich text) Used to exchange files cross-platform. Rtf files are readable by most word processing programs even if the file wasn't created in those programs.
- .bmp: (image) Used for storing digital bitmapped graphics.

<u>Spreadsheets</u>

Historically, a **spreadsheet** has been a bookkeeping document—often found in a ledger with two facing pages and columns and cells to enter information. These are still used in some businesses, especially small businesses, but almost all larger businesses utilize an electronic spreadsheet, which is a software application that organizes and stores data (numeric or text) in tables and allows for analysis. Cells in a spreadsheet are arranged in columns and rows. A commonly-used spreadsheet is Microsoft Excel. Spreadsheets were originally used primarily for budgetary reasons to track income and expenditures, but use has expanded. For example, spreadsheets are used extensively in education to keep track of assignments and grades and to report grades. They are used in research to keep track of results. If the spreadsheet program is part of a software productivity suite (such as Microsoft Office) then information from the spreadsheet can be easily exported into other applications, such as the word processing program.

Social Media

Some medical practices/organizations utilize **social media,** such as blogs, social networks, and websites, to communicate with patients and allow patients to set up appointments, obtain lab results, send messages, and receive messages. Strict protocols should be established for use of social media by healthcare professionals, including who has access, how access is obtained, the types of responses that are appropriate, and methods of dealing with inappropriate comments (such as from an angry patient). Personal social media, such as a personal Facebook account or Twitter account, should never be used to discuss any patient, patient care, or other healthcare-related issues associated with employment as this may violate HIPAA regulations regarding privacy and security and could place the practice/organization at risk for liability. Some healthcare organizations do not permit employees to even mention the place of employment on social media, so the CMAA must review employment policies.

Searching Online Information

Boolean Logic

Boolean logic, developed by the mathematician George Boole in the 1800s is used to search databases and is recognized by most search engines, such as Google. Search is conducted for keywords connected by the operators AND, OR, and NOT. Boolean searching is often used with truncations and wildcards:

- Truncations: "Finan*" provides all words that begin with those letters, such as "finance," "financial" and "financed."
- Wildcards: "m?n" or "m*n" provides "man" and "men."
- AND: "Wound AND antibiotic" produces all documents that contain both words.
- OR: "Wound OR Infect* OR ulcer" produces documents that contain "wound" and either "infect*" or "ulcer." This query is especially useful to search for a number of synonyms or variant spellings. This query may return a large number of documents. OR may be combined with other operators: Wound OR ulcer AND Povidone-iodine
- NOT: Wound AND povidone-iodine NOT antibiotic NOT antimicrobial. NOT is used to exclude keywords.

PICOT

The **PICOT** format is one method of developing appropriate questions to use in searching online information. This method helps clarify the question and necessary information and to identify key words utilized in searching.

P	Patient/ Population	List important characteristics: 35-year-old male with low back pain.
I	Intervention/ Indicator	Explain the desired intervention under consideration: Acupuncture.
C	Comparison/ Control	List other possible interventions or alternatives: Surgery.
O	Outcome	Provide the desired measurable outcomes: Decreased pain levels (from 6-7 to 1-2) and increased mobility.
T	Time	Timeframe (if appropriate)

This format is then used to formulate a question:

- In a 35-year-old male with low back pain, how does acupuncture compared with surgery affect pain levels and mobility?

Based on this question, then the search may be conducted with the following (including synonyms): (Back pain or sciatica) and (acupuncture or surgery) and (pain management or pain-free or pain control).

Blogs and LISTSERV

Blogs (web logs) are online journals that can be set up for free and to which people can comment. Many are personal blogs, but health-related and support group blogs are increasingly available. However, many of the current health-related blogs are set up by consumers rather than healthcare professionals, so information is not always reliable. While blogs are essentially electronic diaries, they can be easily adapted for educational purposes. Blogs can be set up for all types of learners and for stand-alone content or content in support of other classwork. Blogs can contain text, audio, images, and video and can link to other websites and blogs. **LISTSERV™** is a commercial software automated mailing list product that allows users to send an email to multiple users rather than sending individual emails. A free application is available that allows the user to create up to 10 lists of up to 500 individuals, and other companies make similar software applications. These applications are sometimes simply referred to as "listservs," but the term is trademarked.

Social Network Sites

Social network sites are usually Web 2.0 sites. The primary characteristic of a Web 2.0 site is interactivity. Instead of the application being on the individual's computer, it is based on the Internet. Typical Web 2.0 sites include social media (such as Facebook) that allow users to manipulate data and comment as well as YouTube, which allows users to watch videos and upload videos. Commonly used social network sites include:

- LinkedIn is a network designed for professionals and professional communications. Members are able to access information about jobs, current trends, and professional news as well as information about marketing.
- Facebook is an open social media site that is used for personal communications as well as special-interest groups but is less focused on business.
- Twitter allows instant messages to followers. While originally limited to 140 characters, this limitation has been removed.

When initiating a social media site to provide information about a healthcare organization and to allow feedback, the best way of handling feedback from the public is to monitor and censor if inappropriate.

Scanning of Documents

Scanning is a fairly straight-forward procedure that involves placing a document in a scanner and pressing a button that converts the document into a form that can be transmitted to a computer in digital form or can be copied and printed. For instance, scanning is often used to place print documents, such as consultation reports, into electronic health records. However, scanners must be HIPAA compliant, so data must be transmitted under security protocols that prevent unauthorized access. Some scanners store images of scanned documents, so access to such scanners should be password protected and protocols in place for securely deleting files because HIPAA requires that hard drives be wiped of all protected health information. Both before and after scanning, documents must be stored securely and cannot be left unattended. Scanned images should be checked for accuracy before original documents are destroyed, usually by shredding.

Faxing

Faxing is often used to send documents, such as patient records and consultation reports, over the telephone line because it is fast and efficient. However, sending records by fax can make documents vulnerable to HIPAA violations, so some precautions should be used:

- Double-check the correct fax number. If calling to ask for a fax number, always repeat the number to ensure it was received correctly.
- Telephone the intended recipient in advance so that they are expecting the fax and can remove it from the fax machine immediately. Ask the recipient to verify receipt by a return call, email, or text message.

- Enter the telephone number carefully and check digital display if available to make sure the number is correct. If not, immediately disconnect.
- Include a fax cover sheet that indicates the documents are confidential and instructs the recipient who receives the documents in error to immediately destroy them.

Copiers

Copiers are machines that make one or multiple copies of documents and can enlarge or decrease the size of the copied documents. Many copiers also can be used as scanners. Some copiers are large, but small card copier/scanners are available to copy or scan insurance and/or ID cards. After documents are placed on the copier, the number of copies must be selected as well as the paper size and orientation and color preference. As with scanners, most current models of copiers have a hard drive and some store every document copied or scanned. These machines must be HIPAA compliant and access password protected with protocols in place to delete stored images to prevent unauthorized access. It's important to always check the copier to ensure all documents have been removed when done copying. Documents left by accident in the copier or sitting and waiting to be copied may be accessed by unauthorized people.

Computer Use

Audit Trails

Audit trails are records of activity related to systems and applications and users access and utilization of systems and applications. One system may employ a number of different audit trails. Audit trails are a security tool that allows administrators to track individual users, identify the cause of problems, note data modification and misuse of equipment, and reconstruct computer events. Audit trails can also indicate penetration or attempted penetration. Audit trails include event records and keystroke monitoring, which shows each keystroke entered by a user and the electronic response:

- Audit trails at the system level generally record any logins (including ID, date, time) and devices used and functions.
- Audit trails at the application level monitors activity within the application, including opened files, editing, reading, deleting, and printing.
- Audit trails for users include all activities by the user, such as commands, accessed files, and deletions.

Terms Associated with Computer Use	
Audit trail	Record of computer activity that can trace activity of users.
Backup	A second copy of data that can be archived in case data is lost.
Cloud server	A server that collects information over the Internet and stores the information at a distance.
Cold boot	Starting the computer after it has been powered down.
Database	Electronic collection of related data that can be stored and accessed through queries.
Decryption	Changing text that has been encrypted to a readable form.
Dumb terminal	A computer that lacks a hard drive but is connected to another so that only some activities can be carried out, such as access to software or the Internet.
Encryption	Coding data (such as emails) so that they cannot be read without a decryption code.
Ethernet	A communication system that connects several computers.

Field	Database component that stores a separate piece of data.
Firewall	Software program or device that prevents unauthorized access to computers/networks.
Input device	Device that allows the user to enter data into a computer, such as a keyboard.
Modem	Device that connects to a router to allow access to the Internet.
Port	Interface that allows other devices to be connected to a computer.
Privacy filter	A privacy screen placed over the monitor that allows viewing of information on the screen only if sitting directly in front of the screen.
Resolution	Sharpness/Clearness of an image, depending on the number of pixels displayed.
Search engine	A set of programs, such as Google and Bing, that search the web for information based on a query.
Spyware	An unwanted program that runs in the background of software and collects data without the user's knowledge.
Virus	A software program that attaches to another software program and can spread to other computers if files are transmitted.
ZIP file	A file that has been compressed so that it is smaller for transmission but expands on opening so that data can be sent more quickly.

Basic Medical Terminology

Body Planes and Anatomic Terms

Body planes include:

- Sagittal/Lateral: Vertical plane separating right from left.
- Median/Midsagittal: Sagittal plane at midline (middle) separating the body into equal top and bottom halves.
- Coronal/Frontal: Vertical plane separating anterior (front) from posterior (back).
- Axial/Transverse: Horizontal plane that separates the body into superior (upper) and inferior (lower) parts.

A cross-section is an axial/transverse (horizontal) cut through a tissue specimen or body structure while a longitudinal section is a sagittal or coronal (vertical) cut.

Medial is toward the midline while lateral is away from the midline and to the side. Distal is farthest from the point of reference and proximal is closest. When describing an area of the patient's body, the description should be patient-oriented, using phrases such as "patient's left" and "patient's right" to ensure accurate interpretation.

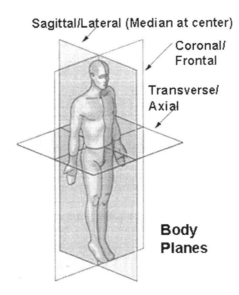

Abdominal Regions

Abdominal regions of the body include:

- A: Right hypochondriac
- B: Epigastric (Epi = on, above)
- C: Left hypochondriac
- D: Right lumbar
- E: Umbilical
- F: Left lumbar
- G: Right iliac

- H: Hypogastric (Hypo = below, beneath, less than normal)
- I: Left iliac

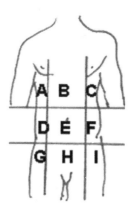

The abdomen may also be divided into 4 quadrants (sections) with the umbilicus (navel) at center: Right upper quadrant (RUQ), right lower quadrant (RLQ), left upper quadrant (LUQ) and left lower quadrant (LLQ). When describing an area of the patient's body, the description should be patient-oriented, using phrases such as "patient's left" and "patient's right" to ensure accurate interpretation.

Anatomic Terms

Term	Meaning
Anterior	Situated toward the front
Posterior	Situated toward the back
Superior	Situated above
Inferior	Situated below
Midline	In the middle
Medial	Situated toward the midline
Lateral	Situated toward the side, away from the midline
Distal	Farthest from the point of reference. When referring to limbs, it means toward the hand or foot.
Proximal	Closest to the point of reference. With limbs, it means toward the elbow/shoulder or knee/hip.
Anteroposterior	From front to back
Posteroanterior	From back to front
Cranial	Toward the head
Caudal	Toward the feet, below another structure
Dorsal	The back of the body
Ventral	The front of the body/ Abdomen
Pronation	Palm/Sole down
Supination	Palm/Sole up

Measurements

Abbreviation	Meaning
cm	centimeter
g, gm	gram
gt	drop
gtt	drops
Kg	kilogram
L	liter
lb	pounds
Mcg	microgram
m	meter
mL	milliliter
mg	milligram
mEq	milliequivalent
Ng	nanogram

Symbols

Symbol	Meaning	Example
/	per	5 mg/kg/hr (5 milligrams per kilogram per hour)
↑	Increase	Temp ↑
↓	Decrease	Pain level ↓
⌀	None, negative	Purulent discharge ⌀
#	Number	Part # 7602
?	Unsure, information needed	Previous vaccinations?
°	Degrees	37° C (centigrade) or 98.6° F (Fahrenheit)
>	greater than	Distance of >3 feet.
→	→ = greater than	
<	less than	slow gait (<0.6 m/second)
←	less than	
+	Positive	
−	negative	

Common Medical Abbreviations

Abbreviation	Meaning
Abd	abdomen
ADL	activities of daily living
AK	above the knee
AMA	against medical advice
ASAP	as soon as possible
BC	birth control
Bx	biopsy
BK	below the knee

- 89 -

Abbreviation	Meaning
BM	bowel movement
BMI	body mass index
BSA	body surface area
CABG	coronary artery bypass graft
CAT/CT	computerized (axial) tomography
CDC	Centers for Disease Control & Prevention
C/O	complaints of
CPAP	continuous positive airway pressure
CPR	cardiopulmonary resuscitation
CXR	chest x-ray
D&C	dilation and curettage
DNR	do not resuscitate
DOA	dead on arrival
DOI	date of injury
Dx	diagnosis
ECG/EKG	electrocardiogram
EEG	electroencephalogram
EENT	eyes, ears, nose, and throat
FF	force fluids
FTND	full-term normal delivery
GSW	gunshot wound
HC	head circumference
HOH	hard of hearing
H&P	history and physical
Hx	history
ICP	intracranial pressure
I&O	intake and output
LBW	low birth weight
MRI	magnetic resonance imaginary
MVA	motor vehicle accident
NB	newborn
N/C	no complaints
NKA	no known allergies
OB	obstetrics
OT	occupational therapy
Pap	Papanicolaou smear
PARA	number of births
PCI	percutaneous coronary intervention
PDR	Physician's Desk Reference
PET	positron emission tomography
PICC	peripherally inserted central catheter
PHI	protected health information
PMI	past medical history
PN	parenteral nutrition
PT	physical therapy
PTA	prior to admission
Px	prognosis

Abbreviation	Meaning
SH	social history
SOAP	subjective, objective, assessment, plan
SOB	short of breath
T&A	tonsillectomy & adenoidectomy
TAB	therapeutic abortion
TEDS	thromboembolic disease stockings
TEE	transesophageal echocardiogram
TENS	transcutaneous electrical nerve stimulation
TO	telephone order
TURP	transurethral resection of the prostate
Tx	treatment
US	ultrasound
VO	verbal order
WNL	within normal limits
W/U	workup

Common Abbreviations and Symbols for Medical Orders

Abbreviation/Symbol	Meaning	Abbreviation/Symbol	Meaning
ac	before meals	w or c̄	with
pc	after meals	w/o or s̄	without
BID	twice daily	BP	blood pressure
TID	3 X daily	TPR	temp., pulse, & resp.
QID	4 X daily	VS	vital signs (BP, TPR)
QOD	every other day	ol or os	left eye
HS	hour of sleep	od	right eye
q	every (q 4 hr)	ou	each eye
c/o	complains of	IM	intramuscular
hr/hrs	hour/hours	SQ	subcutaneous
Rx	treatment, prescription	IV	intravenous
NPO	nothing per mouth)	ID	intradermal
NG	nasogastric	PO	by mouth (*per os*)
R/O	rule out	stat	immediately
ROM	range of motion	prn	as needed

Abbreviations and Acronyms for Common Diagnoses

Abbreviations/Acronyms	Meaning
ADD	attention deficit disorder
ADHD	attention deficit hyperactivity disorder
AF	atrial fibrillation
AHD	atherosclerotic heart disease
AIDS	acquired immune deficiency syndrome
ALL	acute lymphocytic/lymphoblastic leukemia
ALS	amyotrophic lateral sclerosis

Abbreviations/Acronyms	Meaning
AML	acute myeloblastic/myelocytic leukemia
ARDS	acute respiratory distress syndrome
ASCVD	arteriosclerotic cardiovascular disease
BBB	bundle branch block
BPH	benign prostatic hypertrophy
CA	cancer, carcinoma
CHF	congestive heart failure
CIS	carcinoma in situ
CKD	chronic kidney disease
COPD	chronic obstructive pulmonary disease
CPD	cephalopelvic disproportion
CRF	chronic renal failure
CVA	cerebrovascular accident (stroke)
CVD	cardiovascular disease
DJD	degenerative joint disease
DTs	delirium tremens
DVT	deep vein thrombosis
ED	erectile dysfunction
ESLD	end-stage liver disease
ESRD	end-stage renal disease
FAS	fetal alcohol syndrome
FB	foreign body
FTT	failure to thrive
Fx	Fx
GBD	gallbladder disease
HBV	hepatitis B
HB	hepatitis C
HF	heart failure
HIV	human immunodeficiency virus
HOH	hard of hearing
HPV	human papillomavirus
HTN	hypertension
IBS	irritable bowel syndrome
IDDM	insulin-dependent diabetes mellitus
LVH	left ventricular hypertrophy
MD	muscular dystrophy, manic depression
MI	myocardial infarction
MVP	mitral valve prolapse
NAD	no acute distress
NIDDM	non-insulin-dependent diabetes mellitus
OA	osteoarthritis
OAG	open-angle glaucoma
OBS	organic brain syndrome
OCD	obsessive-compulsive disorder
PA	pernicious anemia
PAT	paroxysmal atrial contraction
PCD	polycystic disease

Abbreviations/Acronyms	Meaning
PDA	patent ductus arteriosus
PE	pulmonary edema/embolism
PID	pelvic inflammatory disease
PKU	phenylketonuria
PMS	premenstrual syndrome
PTSD	post-traumatic stress disease
PUD	peptic ulcer disease
PVC	premature ventricular contraction
RA	rheumatoid arthritis
SAB	spontaneous abortion
SAH	subarachnoid hemorrhage
SBE	shortness of breath on exertion
SC	sickle cell
SIDS	sudden infant death syndrome
SLE	systemic lupus erythematosus
STD	sexually-transmitted disease
SVT	supraventricular tachycardia
URI	upper respiratory infection
UTI	urinary tract infection
VD	vomiting/diarrhea, venereal disease
VT	ventricular tachycardia
VF	ventricular fibrillation

Common Laboratory Abbreviations

Abbreviation	Meaning	Abbreviation	Meaning
A1c/HgA1c	Hemoglobin A1c	GC	gonorrhea culture
ABG	arterial blood gases	GFR	glomerular filtration rate
BG	blood glucose	GH	growth hormone
BMP	basal metabolic panel	GTT	glucose tolerance test
BS	blood sugar	Hb/Hgb	hemoglobin
BUN	blood, urea, nitrogen	hCG	human chorionic gonadotropin hormone
Ca	calcium	HDL	high density lipoproteins
CBC	complete blood count	Hct	hematocrit
Chem	chemistry	H&H	hemoglobin & hematocrit.
Chol	cholesterol	INR	internal normalized ratio
Cl	chloride	K/KCL	potassium (chloride)
CMH	comprehensive metabolic panel	LDH	lactic dehydrogenase
CPK	creatinine phosphokinase	LFT	liver function tests
CrCl	creatinine clearance	LH	luteinizing hormone
CPK	Creatinine phosphokinase	Mag	magnesium
C&S	culture & sensitivities	Na/NaCl	sodium (chloride)
CSF	cerebrospinal fluid	O&P	ova and parasites
Diff	differential	P	phosphorus
EBV	Epstein-Barr virus	PT	prothrombin time

Abbreviation	Meaning	Abbreviation	Meaning
ELISA	enzyme-linked immunosorbent assay	PTT	partial thromboplastin time
ESR	erythrocyte sedimentation rate	Qns	quantity not sufficient
ETOH	ethyl alcohol	RBC	red blood cells
FBS	fasting blood sugar	Sp. gr.	specific gravity
Fe	iron	UA	urinalysis
FS	frozen section	UC	urine culture
FSH	follicle stimulating hormone	WBC	white blood cells

Prefixes, Suffixes, and Roots

Medical words are comprised of prefixes, suffixes, and roots in various combinations. Prefixes are found at the beginning of a word and suffixes at the end. Roots may be found at the beginning (if there is no suffix) or in the middle but generally require a suffix to end the word. More than one root may occur in a word. The meaning is not always completely literal. For example, the word *antibiotic* literally means "pertaining to against life" but it captures the essence of the meaning, "a medication that destroys microorganisms." The letter *o* (most commonly) or *i* is often used as a combining form:

Word	Prefix	Root	Suffix
anemia	an- (without, less, not)	em (blood)	-ia (condition)

The meaning of most medical words is derived by starting with the suffix and then the prefix and root; thus, anemia means literally a condition with less blood. All words must have at least one root. Gastroenterology is the study of the stomach and intestines.

Word	Root	o	Root	o	Suffix
gastroenterology	gastr- (stomach)	o	-enter- (intestines)	o	-logy (study of)

Electroencephalogram is a record of the electrical activity of the brain.

Word	Root	o	Root	o	Suffix
electroencephalogram	electr- (electricity)	o	-encephal- (brain)	o	-gram (record)

Common Prefixes

Prefix	Meaning	Examples
hyper-	Enlarged, excessive, high	Hypertrophy (enlarged tissue), hyperemesis (excessive vomiting), hyperactive (over-active), hypertension (condition of high blood pressure)
hypo-	Under, beneath, low	Hypoglycemia (low blood sugar), hypotension (low blood pressure), hypoxia (low oxygen)
eu-	Good, normal	Euthanasia (good death), euthyroid (normal functioning thyroid)
pre-	Before	Preoperative (before operation)
post-	After, behind	Postoperative (after operation)
peri-	About, around	Peritonsillar (about the tonsils), perivascular (around a vessel)
poly-	Many	Polyarthritis (inflammation of many joints)
retro-	Behind	Retroperitoneal (behind the peritoneum)

Prefix	Meaning	Examples
endo-	Within, in	Endocarditis (infection within the heart), endometritis (infection within the uterus), endocrine (gland that secretes inside)
exo-	Outside of, without	Exocrine (gland that secretes outside, such as to the skin), exogenous (originating outside)
ab-	Away from	Abduction (process of movement away from the body)
ad-	Toward	Adduction (process of movement toward the body)
anti-	Against, opposed to	Antibiotic (literally: pertaining to opposed to life), antisocial (against society)
auto	Self	Autocytolysis (self-destruction of cells), autograft (graph from one part of a person's body to another)
hemi-	Half	Hemiplegia (condition of paralysis of half of the body)
inter-	Between	Intercostal (between the ribs)
intra-	Within	Intraspinal (within the spine), intraoral (within the mouth)
brady-	Slow	Bradycardia (condition of slow heart)
tachy	Rapid, fast	Tachycardia (condition of rapid heart)
trans-	Across	Transplacental (across the placenta)

Common Roots

Root	Meaning	Root	Meaning	Root	Meaning
abdomin	abdomen	enceph/al	brain	pnea	breathing
aden	gland	enter	intestines	pulmon	lung
alges	pain	ede	swelling	rect	rectum
arth	joint	gastr	stomach	sanguin	blood
arter/i	artery	gyn	female	sept	infection
brach/i	arm	hem/hemat/em	blood	thorac	chest
carcin	cancer	my	muscle	trich	hair
card/i	heart	nas	nose	vas	vessel
cephal	head	neuro	nerve	ven	vein
chole	bile, gall	ophthalm	eye	viscer	viscera
col	colon	opt	vision, sight	voc	voice
cyst	cyst, bladder	or	mouth	xer	dry
cyt	cell	oste	bone		
derm	skin	ot	ear		

Common Suffixes

Suffix	Meaning	Examples
-gram	Picture, record	Electrocardiogram (record of the electrical activity of the heart)
-graph	Instrument for recording	Electrocardiograph (instrument for recording the electrical activity of the heart)
-cytosis	Increase in cells	Leukocytosis (increased white blood cells), thrombocytosis (increased platelets)
-penia	Decrease in cells	Leukopenia (decreased white blood cells), neutropenia (decreased neutrophils), thrombocytopenia (decreased platelets)
-otomy	Incision	Colectomy (incision of the colon)

Suffix	Meaning	Examples
-ectomy	Surgical removal	Colectomy (surgical removal of the colon), tonsillectomy (surgical removal of the tonsils)
-stomy	Surgical creation of body opening	Colostomy (creation of an opening into the colon), tracheostomy (creation of an opening into the trachea)
-scopy	Examination with a scope	Bronchoscopy (examination of the bronchi with a scope)
-megaly	Enlargement	Hepatomegaly (enlargement of the liver), splenomegaly (enlargement of the spleen)
-ac, -ic, -ary,- al	Pertaining to	Cardiac (pertaining to the heart), rhythmic (pertaining to rhythm), solitary (pertaining to being alone), renal (pertaining to the kidney)
-ist	Person	Cardiologist (person who studies the heart), pathologist (person who studies disease)
-itis	Inflammation	Cholecystitis (inflammation of the gall bladder), cystitis (inflammation of the bladder)
-lysis	destruction	Cytolysis (condition of destruction of cells), hemolysis destruction of blood)
-sis	Condition of	Arteriosclerosis (condition of hardening of the arteries)
-oma	tumor	Neuroma (tumor of the nerves), lymphoma (tumor of the lymph system)
-tion	Process of, act of, result of	Elongation (process of becoming longer)
-pathy	disease	Neuropathy (disease of the nerves), myopathy (disease of the muscles)
-phobia	Condition of fear of	Herpetophobia (condition of fear of snakes), agoraphobia (literally: condition of fear of the marketplace)
-plegia	Condition of paralysis	Quadriplegia (condition of paralysis of four [limbs])

Interpretation of Signs and Symbols

Sign/Symbol	Interpretation
	Flame: Includes flammable materials and gases and those that are self-heating or self-reactive.
	Corrosion: Includes substances that can cause skin burns, metal corrosion, and eye damage.
	Health hazard: Includes carcinogens, toxic substances, and respiratory irritants.

Sign/Symbol	Interpretation
	Poison: Includes materials, gases, or substances that are extremely toxic and may result in death or severe illness.
	Irritant: Includes material, gases, or substances that are irritants to skin, eyes, and/or respiratory tract, acutely toxic, or have a narcotic effect.
	Biohazard: Includes biological substances, such as body fluids, that pose a threat to humans. Appears on sharps containers that hold contaminated needles.

Basic Spelling and Pronunciation Guidelines

Medical terminology utilizes many words derived from Greek or Latin, so spelling and pronunciation follow predictable patterns.

Spelling	Sounds like	Examples
c (before a, o, or u)	K (kitten)	cavity, coma, cardiac
c (before e, i, or y)	S (sat)	cephalic, circulation, cytology
ch	K (kitten)	cholesterol, cholecystitis, chlorine (Exception: choke)
g (before a, o, or u)	G (give)	gastric, gonad, Guillain-Barré
g (before e or i)	J (jar)	generic, genitals, gingival
i (used to make plural)	I ("eye")	bronchus/bronchi, embolus/emboli, fundus/fundi
ph	F (fat)	lymph, phlebitis, phobia
pn	N (no)	pneumonia, pneumothorax
ps	S (sat)	psychology, pseudoencephalitis, pseudomonas
pt	T (to)	ptosis, ptyalism, pterygium
rh or rrh	R (rat)	rhythm, diarrhea, dysrhythmia, hemorrhoid
X (first letter of word)	Z (zoo)	xerosis, xeroderma, xanthine (Exception: x-ray)

Singular and Plural Forms

Plural rule	Singular	Plural
-a to -ae	vertebra, axilla, sclera	vertebrae, axillae, sclerae
-um to -a	bacterium, diverticulum	bacteria, diverticula
-us to -i	thrombus, embolus, bronchus	thrombi, emboli, bronchi (Exceptions: corpus/corpora, meatus/meatus, viscus/viscera, plexus, plexuses)
-is to -es	metastasis, testis, diagnosis	metastases, testes, diagnoses (Exceptions: epididymis/epididymides, femur/femora, iris/irides)
-ma or -oma to -mata	carcinoma, fibroma, condyloma	carcinomata, fibromata, condylomata (Note: simply adding -s is now also acceptable)
-ax, -ix, and -yx to -ces	thorax, appendix, calyx	thoraces, appendices, calyces
-nx to -nges	pharynx, phalanx	pharynges, phalanges

Plural rule	Singular	Plural
-y after a consonant to -ies	artery, ovary, bronchoscopy	arteries, ovaries, bronchoscopies
Irregular	Cornu, vas, pons	Cornua, vasa, pontes

Disabilities

A **disability** is an impairment that limits a person's ability to function in some way. Disabilities may be mild or severe and may be obvious or hidden. For Social Security or SSI, specific criteria must be met for a patient to be classified as disabled. Disabilities include:

Disability	Description
Physical	Defect in body function, such as may occur with chronic conditions, such as osteoarthritis in the knees, amputations, or paralysis.
Sensory	Vision and hearing deficits as well as impaired sense of taste and smell, touch, and/or balance
Intellectual	Cognitive impairment, such as may occur with traumatic brain injury, Alzheimer's disease, and intellectual disabilities.
Mental	Mental health disorder that impairs functioning, such as schizophrenia, severe depression, and bipolar disease.
Neurodevelopmental/ Developmental	Impaired ability to socialize and communicate, such as with autism spectrum disorder, Rett syndrome, and ADHD or impaired growth and development, such as with spina bifida.

Bones of the Skeleton

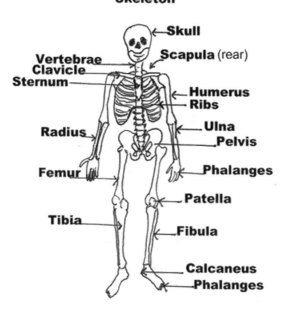

- 98 -

Cranial and Facial Nerves

Cranial Nerves	Facial Nerves (Cranial nerve VII)
I. Olfactory: Smell. II. Optic: Vision. III. Oculomotor IV. Trochlear: Eye muscle, upward movement. V. Trigeminal: Chewing, sensory perception. VI. Abducens: Eye movement, lateral movement. VII. Facial: Expressions, tears, taste, saliva. VIII. Vestibular: Balance and hearing. IX. Glossopharyngeal: Taste, mouth sensation. X. Vagus: Swallowing, gag reflex. XI. Spinal accessory: Shoulder muscle movement. XII. Hypoglossal: Tongue.	 **Facial nerves** Temporal Zygomatic Buccal Post. auricular Mandibular Cervical

Sexually-Transmitted Diseases

Disease	Characteristics
Gonorrhea	Caused by the bacterium *Neisseria gonorrhoeae*. Transmission through anal, oral, or vaginal sex. Infection may pass to newborn during birth, causing gonorrheal eye infection and blindness unless eye prophylaxis provided.
Chlamydia	Most common STD in the US. Caused by bacterium *Chlamydia trachomatis*. Transmission through anal, oral or vaginal sex. Often occurs with gonorrhea. May be asymptomatic but can lead to pelvic inflammatory disease (females) and epididymitis (males).
Syphilis	Bacterial infection with *Treponema pallidum*, transmission through oral, anal, or vaginal sex and needle sharing. Symptoms vary depending on stage. Can transmit to fetus, causing birth defects.
Herpes simples 2	Transmitted though oral, anal, or vaginal sex. Virus enters nerve endings, travels to the nerve ganglion, and stays dormant until reactivated by stress, immunosuppression, menstruation, sunburn, illness, or other triggers.
Human papillomavirus (HPV)	Transmission through vaginal, anal, or oral sex. May invade mucosal tissue, causing genital warts and/or changes that can lead to cervical or penile cancer.

Common Childhood Diseases for Which Children Are Vaccinated

Disease	Characteristics

Mumps	Viral disease that causes fever and swollen parotid glands but can cause deafness, meningitis, and swelling of the testicles. Mumps is spread through contact with saliva or aerosolized droplets from someone infected. MMR (measles, mumps, rubella) vaccination available.
Rubella (German measles)	Viral disease that can cause rash, fever, arthritis, encephalitis, and death. Rubella can cause a woman who is pregnant to miscarry or deliver a child with serious birth defects. Transmission is through airborne droplets. MMR vaccination available.
Rubeola (measles)	Viral disease characterized by fever and rash but can cause serious morbidity and death. It is highly infectious by droplets 4 days before and 4 days after onset of rash. MMR vaccination available.
Varicella (chicken pox)	Caused by the varicella zoster virus, resulting in fever, rash, and itching, but it can cause skin infections, pneumonia, and neurological damage. After infection, the virus retreats to the nerves by the spinal cord and can reactivate years later, causing herpes zoster (shingles), a significant cause of morbidity in adults. Varicella vaccination available.

Vaccines

Vaccine	Description
MMR	Provides immunity to measles, mumps, and rubella
Varicella	Provides immunity to chicken pox.
Meningococcal polysaccharide vaccine	Provides immunity to meningitis for children 2-10.
Meningococcal conjugate	Provides immunity to meningitis for children >11 who have not received Meningococcal polysaccharide vaccine.
Heptavalent pneumococcal conjugate (PCV-7) (Prevnar)	Provides immunity to children <2 or up to 5 if at high risk against *Streptococcus pneumoniae* to protect against invasive pneumococcal disease, such as pneumonia, otitis media, bacteremia, and meningitis.
Pneumococcal polysaccharide-23	Provides immunity against 23 types pneumococcal bacteria, which can cause pneumonia, for adults ≥65 and children ≥ at high risk.
Haemophilus influenzae type b (HIB)	Provides immunity to infection that can cause severe respiratory infections, pneumonia, meningitis, and pericarditis, for children ≤5.
Influenza	Provides immunity against annual flu for those 6 months and older.
Herpes zoster (Shingrix or Zostavax)	Provides immunity against herpes zoster (shingles) infection for adults ≥50.
HPV	Provides immunity to human papillomavirus for males and females ages 9 to 45. Recommended at ages 11-12.
Hepatitis B	Provides immunity to hepatitis B infection. First injection administered shortly after birth.

Fractures

Types of Fractures

	Transverse: Usually occur in long bones and are at risk of displacement unless splinted to prevent movement. Most often occur from direct impact, such as sports injuries. May suggest abuse if they occur in small children.
	Comminuted: Usually result from high impact trauma, such as with motor vehicle accidents, and are more common in older adults or those with weakened bones. This fracture is very painful and often accompanied by swelling and muscle spasms.
	Spiral: Common in toddlers who fall on extended leg, breaking tibia, but may also occur with abuse in small children as a result on jerking or twisting an extremity (usually the arm).
	Displaced: Pose risk of damage to surrounding tissue, including nerves and blood vessels, and may lead to an open fracture if not properly splinted. Usually deformity is evident.
	Greenstick: Most common in children whose bones are less hard and are usually quite painful but without deformity.

Orthopedic Terms

Term	Meaning
Amputation	Surgical or traumatic removal of a body part, such as an amputation of the leg.
Bursitis	Inflammation of bursae (fluid-filled sacs that cushion joints).
Dislocation	Displacement of a part (generally a bone from a socket), such as a dislocation of the elbow or shoulder.
Fracture	Break in a part, primarily a bone or tooth.
Kyphosis	Convex curvature of the vertebrae.
Lordosis	Concave curvature of the vertebrae.
Rupture	Tear and separation, such as a ruptured Achille's tendon.
Scoliosis	Twisting or curvature of the vertebrae.
Sprain	Wrenching of a joint with damage (tearing, stretching) to the ligaments (which connect bones), such as a sprained ankle.
Strain	Overstretched or torn muscle, such as a hamstring strain.
Tendinitis	Inflammation of the tendons, which attach muscles to bones.

Common Soft Tissue Injury Terms

Injury	Characteristics
Abrasion	Painful superficial scraping of outermost layer of skin. Little or no bleeding.
Avulsion	Skin and underlying soft tissue is torn away, such as with degloving injury, from any part of the body although lower extremity injury is most common. Bleeding may be severe, especially if vessels are torn or exposed.
Blast injury	Involves varying degrees of soft tissue injury and sometimes amputations, fractures, impalements, traumatic brain injuries, ruptured eardrum, pulmonary injury, perforated bowel, and burns.
Foreign body in eye	Patient has pain, tearing, redness, blurred or impaired vision from dirt, dust, chemical or other material in eye(s).

Injury	Characteristics
Impaled object	Penetrating object remains in wound.
Laceration	Cut or break in skin from impact with sharp object. Bleeding may vary from mild to severe.
Puncture	Wound from impact with sharp pointed object (knife, bullet) may exhibit little external bleeding but major internal bleeding and soft tissue damage. Exit wound may be present.

Common Obstetrics/Pregnancy Terms

Term	Meaning
Abruptio placentae	Placenta prematurely detaches, partially or completely, from the uterus.
Breech presentation	Fetus enters birth canal with buttock or feet first. Frank breech (buttocks presentation with legs extended upward) is most common, but single or double footling breech or complete breech (buttocks presentation with legs flexed) can occur.
Dilation	Stretching and opening of the cervix to allow birth of infant, estimated in centimeters.
Effacement	Thinning of the cervix in preparation for birth of infant.
Hyperemesis gravidarum	Severe nausea, vomiting, and dehydration associated with pregnancy.
Placenta previa	Placenta implants over or near the internal cervical opening. Implantation may be complete (covering the entire opening), partial, or marginal (to the edge of the cervical opening).
Pre-eclampsia	High blood pressure, protein in urine, and swelling during pregnancy. Can lead to eclampsia (seizures and death).
Preterm labor	Labor between weeks 20 to 37.
Prolapsed cord	The umbilical cord precedes the fetus in the birth canal and becomes entrapped by the descending fetus.
Gravida	Any pregnancy (including present) regardless of duration/outcome.
Nulligravida	A woman who has never been pregnant.
Primigravida	A woman with her first pregnancy.
Multigravida	A woman in her $\geq 2^{nd}$ pregnancy.
Para	Delivery of live or stillborn fetus/neonate >20 weeks gestation.
Nullipara	Woman who has not given birth >20 weeks gestation
Primipara	A woman who has given birth, live or stillborn, one time >20 weeks gestation.
Multipara	A woman who has given birth, live or stillborn, ≥ 2 times >20 weeks gestation.
Grand multipara	A woman who has given birth, live or stillborn, ≥ 5 times >20 weeks gestation.
Term	38 to 48 weeks duration of pregnancy.
Gestation	Number of weeks since the first day of last menstrual period (LMP)>
Abortion	Death of fetus <20 weeks' gestation.
Stillbirth	Death of fetus >20 weeks' gestation.

Antihypertensives and Cardiac Medications

Term	Meaning
Angiotensin-converting enzymes (ACE inhibitors)	ACEIs lower BP by inhibiting an enzyme that causes vessels to constrict, resulting in vasodilation. Include benazepril, captopril, and enalapril.
Angiotensin II receptor blockers (ARBs)	ARBs lower BP by blocking an enzyme (angiotensin II) from causing vessels to constrict, resulting in vasodilation. Include irbesartan, losartan, and valsartan.
Antiarrhythmics/ Antidysrhythmics	Treat abnormal heart rates and rhythms caused by irregular electrical activity. Include amiodarone (Cordarone), flecainide, procainamide (Procan), propafenone (Rythmol) and tocainide.
Beta-adrenergic blocker (BBs)	"Beta blockers" block epinephrine (adrenaline) effects to lower BP. Include atenolol, metoprolol, nadolol, and propranolol.
Calcium channel blockers (CCBs)	CCBs lower BP and relieve angina and irregular heartbeats by preventing calcium from building up in the cells of the heart and blood vessels. Include amlodipine (Norvasc). Diltiazem nicardipine, nifedipine, and verapamil.
Digitalis glycosides/ Digoxin	Increases strength of heart and control rate and rhythm, often used for congestive heart failure.
Diuretics	"Water pills" prevent fluid retention and treat high BP. Include hydrochlorothiazide, chlorthalidone, furosemide, and bumetanide.

Common Classes of Medications

Medication	Purpose	Examples
Analgesics	Control pain	May include narcotics, such as morphine or codeine, or OTC medications, such as acetaminophen and aspirin.
Antibiotics	Treat bacterial infections	Include aminoglycosides (gentamicin, tobramycin), penicillins (amoxicillin), cephalosporins (cephalexin), fluoroquinolones (ciprofloxacin, levofloxacin), macrolides (erythromycin, azithromycin), sulfonamides (trimethoprim), and tetracyclines (doxycycline).
Anticholinergics	Treat overactive bladder, incontinence, & reduce secretions	Oxybutynin (Ditropan), atropine, scopolamine, tolterodine (Detrol),
Anticonvulsants/ Antiepileptics	Prevent seizures	Include carbamazepine, valproate, clonazepam, phenobarbital, phenytoin (Dilantin), topiramate, pregabalin, and gabapentin (Neurontin).
Anticoagulants	Blood thinners, prevent blood clots	Include heparin, warfarin (Coumadin), aspirin, rivaroxaban, dabigatran, apixaban, edoxaban, enoxaparin,

Medication	Purpose	Examples
Antidepressants	Treat depression	Include tricyclic antidepressants (amitriptyline, imipramine, nortriptyline), SSRIs (fluoxetine, sertraline citalopram, paroxetine).
Antidiabetics	Treat type 1 and 2 diabetes	Include metformin, sulfonylureas (glipizide, glimepiride), meglitinides (repaglinide, nateglinide), thiazolidinediones (rosiglitazone, pioglitazone), DPP-4 inhibitors (sitagliptin, linagliptin), and GLP-1 receptor agonists (exenatide, liraglutide), and SGLT2 inhibitors (canagliflozin, and dapagliflozin). Various types of insulin (used primarily for type 1 diabetes) include short-acting (Humulin R, Novolin R), rapid-acting (Humalog, NovoLog, Apidra), intermediate acting (Humulin N/NPH, Novolin N/NPH) long-acting (Lantus, Levemir), and premixed preparations.
Antiemetics	Treat nausea & vomiting, motion sickness	Include dimenhydrinate (Dramamine), meclizine (Bonine), metoclopramide (Reglan), and ondansetron (Zofran).
Antifungals	Treat fungal infections	Include amphotericin, clotrimazole, econazole, fluconazole, ketoconazole, and terbinafine.
Antihistamines	Treat allergies	Include diphenhydramine (Benadryl), fexofenadine (Allegra), chlorpheniramine, loratadine (Claritin), and brompheniramine (Dimetane).
89 Antiparkinson/ Dopamine agonists	Treat Parkinson's disease, reduce tremors and slow progression	Include, amantadine, apomorphine, tyrosine hydroxylase, anticholinergic drugs, levodopa, carbidopa, ropinirole (Requip), and pramipexole (Mirapex), carbidopa/levodopa (Sinemet).
Antitussives	Cough medication	Include benzonatate, codeine, and dextromethorphan
Antivirals	Treat viral infections	Include peramivir (Rapivab), zanamivir (Relenza), and oseltamivir phosphate (Tamiflu).
Chemotherapeutic agents	Used to treat cancer, curative and palliative	Includes a wide range of drugs, such as methotrexate, vincristine, 5-fluorouacil, oxaliplatin, cisplatin, cyclophosphamide, doxorubicin, docetaxel, vinblastine, and epirubicin.
Non-steroidal anti-inflammatory drugs (NSAIDS)	Reduce pain and inflammation	Include aspirin, ibuprofen, naproxen, nabumetone, celecoxib (Celebrex), piroxicam (Feldene), indomethacin (Indocin), meloxicam (Mobic), and sulindac (Clinoril).

Medication	Purpose	Examples
Psychotherapeutic agents/psychotropics	Used to treat psychotic mental disorders, such as schizophrenia and bipolar disease	Include atypical antipsychotics, such as olanzapine (Zyprexa), clozapine (Clozaril), quetiapine (Seroquel), risperidone (Risperdal), aripiprazole (Abilify), and pimavanserin (Nuplazid). Also includes phenothiazine antipsychotics, such as chlorpromazine (Thorazine), fluphenazine (Prolixin) and thioridazine (Mellaril).

Common Medications to Treat HIV/AIDS

Medication	Description
Non-nucleoside reverse transcriptase inhibitors (NNRTIs),	Include delavirdine (Rescriptor), efavirenz (Sustiva), etravirine (Intelence), and nevirapine (Viramune) bind to reverse transcriptase and disable it. Reverse transcriptase is a protein required for HIV replication.
Nucleoside reverse transcriptase inhibitors (NRTIs	Include abacavir (Ziagen), abacavir (Epzicom), didanosine (Videx), zidovudine (AZT), tenofovir (Viread), lamivudine (Epivir). These are defective versions of building blocks necessary for replication. When HIV binds to the defective version, it is unable to complete replication.
Protease inhibitors	Disable the protein protease, which HIV requires in order to replicate. PIs include amprenavir (Agenerase), indinavir (Crixivan), nelfinavir (Viracept), saquinavir (Invirase), ritonavir (Norvir), atazanavir sulfate (ATV), Fosamprenavir calcium (Lexiva), tipranavir (TPV), darunavir (Prezista), raltegravir (Isentress) and dolutegravir (Tivicay).
Fusion inhibitors	Include enfuvirtide (Fuzeon) and maraviroc (Selzentry), entry inhibitors that prevent HIV from infecting CD4 cells.

Terms Associated with Physiology of Breathing

Term	Meaning
Tidal volume	Normal volume of gas inhaled during one respiration cycle (approximately 500 mL in a healthy adult).
Inspiratory reserve volume	The volume of air inhaled above tidal volume during forced deep inhalation (up to 3000 mL)
Dead space	Volume of inhaled gas that does not take part in gas exchange.
Alveolar dead space	Volume of alveoli that are ventilated but not perfused.
Vital capacity	Maximum volume of gas that can be forcefully exhaled from the lungs following a full inhalation.
Minute volume	Volume of gas expelled from the lungs in one minute. (Respiratory rate X tidal volume.)
Residual volume	Volume of gas remaining in the lungs after one full forced exhalation.
Total lung capacity	Vital capacity plus residual volume, total volume the lungs can contain (usually about 6000 mL for adults).
Cellular respiration	Utilization of oxygen and glucose to produce energy at the cell level and the creation of water and carbon dioxide as by-products of metabolism.
Oxygenation	Process by which oxygen molecules bind to hemoglobin in the blood.

Terms Associated with Breath Sounds

Term	Meaning
Vesicular	Normal low-pitched sound over lung bases and most lung fields.
Broncho-vesicular	Medium-pitched sound heard over main bronchi. Duration the same in expiration and inspiration.
Bronchial	Normal high-pitched loud sound heard over trachea. Expiratory sound is as long or longer than inspiratory. Abnormal if heard over lung bases.
Rales (crackles)	High-pitched crackles usually heard at end of expiration in lung bases indicating fluid in the alveoli. May be fine or coarse.
Rhonchi	Deep rumbling sound may be high-pitched and sibilant (whistling) or low-pitched and sonorous (snoring) caused by constricted airways or large amounts of secretions in airways. More pronounced on expiration.
Wheezes	High or low-pitched whistling or musical sounds most pronounced on expiration. Often indicate asthma or foreign body obstruction.
Stridor	Crowing sound caused by inflammation and swelling or larynx and trachea. Common finding in croup (associated with cough).
Grunts	Indicates respiratory distress in newborn.
Friction rub	Grating sound heard over area of lungs where pleura are inflamed.

Herbal Products

Herbal Products	Description
Acai	Used for weight loss, to lower cholesterol, to treat erectile dysfunction and to delayed aging, but there is little evidence to support its use. May interfere with MRI.
Black cohosh	Used to relieve symptoms associated with menopause, such as heat flashes and night sweats. Black cohosh contains substances similar to estrogen, phytoestrogens.
Echinacea	Used to prevent and treat colds and flu but use is not supported by scientific studies.
Flaxseed	Used for many reasons (heart disease, high triglyceride levels, hypertension, coronary artery disease, systemic lupus erythematosus) but it appears to be most effective for constipation because of high fiber and oil content.
Garlic	Used to treat heart disease, diabetes, and infections and to reduce risk of cancer. High intake may result in some anticoagulant effect. Garlic may provide some benefit and is relatively safe.
Ginseng	Used to lower blood pressure, regulate blood glucose, and improve the immune system, but may cause diarrhea, insomnia, and other adverse effects.
Gingko biloba	Used to improve memory, reduce anxiety and improve circulation and for a variety of other reasons. Studies have yielded inconsistent evidence of effectiveness.
Glucosamine & chondroitin	Used to relieve arthritis and joint pain. Some studies suggest that it may have some beneficial effect but others show it to be no better than a placebo.

Herbal Products	Description
Melatonin	Used to treat jet lag, insomnia, dementia, and cancer, but there is no evidence that it is effective for dementia or cancer. It appears to be most effective for sleep disorders.
St. John's wort	Used to treat depression. Scientific studies indicate that it may be effective only for mild depression and not severe. It interferes with the action of many drugs, including antidepressants, cyclosporine, warfarin, digoxin, and birth control pills.

Medical Specialists

Physician	Specializes in...
Allergist	diagnosis and treatment of allergies.
Anesthesiologist	administration of anesthesia during surgical and/or diagnostic procedures.
Cardiologist	care and treatment of the heart and circulatory system.
Geneticist	the study of genetics and the genetic basis of disease.
Gynecologist	the care, surgery, and treatment of the female reproductive system.
Hematologist	care and treatment of those with diseases of the blood.
Hospitalist	the care and treatment of hospitalized patients.
Internist	comprehensive care of medical patients, especially those with chronic disease.
Nephrologist	care, treatment, and surgery of those with kidney disease
Neurosurgeon	surgical procedures of the brain, nerves, and spinal cord.
Neurologist	care and treatment of patients with disorders of the brains, nerves, and spinal cord.
Obstetrician	the care and treatment of women who are pregnant. Usually also a gynecologist.
Physician	Specializes in...
Ophthalmologist	the care, treatment, and surgery of conditions of the eye.
Orthopedist	the care, treatment and surgery of musculoskeletal system disorders
Otolaryngologist	the care, treatment, and surgery of the ears, nose, and throat.
Pathologist	the causes of disease, studying cells, tissue, and organs rather providing direct care.
Pediatrician	the care and treatment of children.
Physiatrist	physical medicine and rehabilitation, care of those with disabilities.
Psychiatrist	the care and treatment of those with mental illness.
Pulmonologist	the care and treatment of those with lung disease.
Radiologist	imaging used to detect disease/abnormalities.
Rheumatologist	care and treatment of those with rheumatic diseases or conditions with generalized inflammation and pain and stiffness of muscles and joints.
Urologist	the care, treatment, and surgery of the urinary tract.

Medicolegal Terms/Doctrines

Term/Doctrine	Description
Subpoena	A legal writ (order) requiring a person to come to court, to testify in court, and/or to produce documents or evidence. Failure to do so may result in fine or jailing.
Res ipsa loquitur	("The thing speaks for itself"): The principle of law that allows the use of circumstantial evidence as proof.
Locum tenens	("To substitute for"): Allows one medical professional to serve temporarily in place of another. For example, a physician's practice may be covered by another physician usually for a few days up to 6 months when the first goes on vacation or takes leave. Companies specialize in providing *locums* physicians to work on a contract basis.
Deposition	This is sworn out-of-court witness statements taken under oath, usually in an attorney's office prior to court cases to document what the witness knows and to preserve the statements for use in court.

Practice Test

1. While an answering service takes calls during the night, numerous patients have complained that telephone calls during working hours are often unanswered. The best solution for the office is likely to

    A. hire another staff person to answer the telephone.
    B. ask the answering service to answer after a specified number of rings.
    C. set a voice mail to answer the phone and instruct callers to call back.
    D. have all calls go first to a voicemail system so people can leave messages.

2. If a patient in the waiting room is coughing and no examining rooms are available, the CMAA should

    A. ask the patient to wait outside.
    B. cancel and reschedule the appointment.
    C. ask the patient to cover her mouth when coughing.
    D. provide the patient with a face mask.

3. OSHA's form 301 is used to

    A. describe each workplace death/injury, what actually happened.
    B. list each workplace death/injury.
    C. summarize the number of annual workplace deaths/injuries.
    D. apply for waivers of responsibility.

4. An example of protected health information (PHI) includes

    A. de-identified data regarding types of patients seen by a practice.
    B. a patient's diagnosis.
    C. age range of patients seen by a physician.
    D. sexual abuse of a child.

5. If the physician has indicated on the patient's encounter form that the patient should return for a followup exam in one week but there are no appointment times available for one month, the CMAA should

    A. double-book the patient.
    B. make the appointment in one month.
    C. ask the physician if the patient can wait one month.
    D. schedule the patient by phone after a cancellation.

6. A commonly-used analgesic is

    A. acetaminophen.
    B. furosemide.
    C. penicillin.
    D. atenolol.

7. The distal part of the arm is the part near the

    A, shoulder area.
    B. upper arm
    C. elbow
    D. wrist and hand.

8. When using a copier or scanner for medical records, it is essential to
    A. place a basket near the machine to hold records waiting to be copied or scanned.
    B. make only a single copy of a record at a time.
    C. remove stored information from memory to prevent unauthorized access.
    D. check the printer for equipment for ink when finished.

9. If a new patient calls for an appointment and states that she has been experiencing heavier than usual periods with cramping for the past 3 months, the type of appointment would be categorized as
    A. urgent, acute problem/illness.
    B. new, non-urgent problem/illness.
    C. routine.
    D. physical exam.

10. The ethical principles that states that actions should be carried out for the good of the patient is
    A. beneficence.
    B. maleficence.
    C. justice.
    D. autonomy.

11. If three patients cancel appointments for the same morning, the best solution is to
    A. leave the times free in case other patients call for appointments.
    B. block out free time for the physician and staff.
    C. reschedule afternoon patients to the free times so staff finishes early.
    D. call those on the list for wanting an earlier appointment.

12. The type of healthcare insurance that pays in the form of predetermined payments for loss or damages rather than for healthcare services is
    A. liability insurance.
    B. no-fault auto insurance.
    C. indemnity insurance.
    D. accident and health insurance.

13. The vertical plane that separates anterior from posterior is the
    A. coronal/frontal.
    B. sagittal/lateral plane.
    C. median/midsagittal plane.
    D. axial/transverse.

14. If the appointment matrix shows the following, what is the best time to schedule a new patient who calls at 8:00 AM on June 6 for an appointment to assess increasing edema (swelling) of the feet and mild shortness of breath?

Dr. Jones		
Hr.	June 6	June 7
8:00	Mrs. Smith—BP check	Staff meeting
8:10		" "
8:20	Miss Black--UTI	
8:30	" " " "	Mrs. Smythe--arthritis
8:40		" " " "
8:50	T. Bates—Med. followup	
9:00		S. Brown—post-op check
9:10		
9:20	B. Wood—Pap smear	

    A. 8:10 June 6.
    B. 8:20 June 7.
    C. 8:50 June 7.
    D. 9:00 June 6.

15. If a physician informs the CMAA that she would like to have a conference call with three other physicians at 8:30 AM on the following Monday, the first thing the CMAA should do is to

    A. gather all the telephone numbers for the physician.
    B. contact all participants to confirm telephone numbers, date, and time.
    C. offer to take notes during the conference call.
    D. inform other staff members the physician has scheduled a conference call.

16. The percentage of costs that the patient must pay is the

    A. deductible.
    B. copayment.
    C. co-insurance.
    D. cap.

17. The most effective method of decreasing no shows is to

    A. charge a fee for missed appointments.
    B. admonish the patients for missing appointments.
    C. remind the patients of appointments a day or two before.
    D. avoid extended wait times.

18. A patient has come for a blood pressure check but states, "I think this is a waste of time!" When using the SOAP format, this statement would be documented in which section?

    A. Subjective.
    B. Objective
    C. Assessment.
    D. Plan.

19. If the physician has given the patient directions that state "Eye drops--gtt ii OD TID" and the patient asks what it means, the CMAA would reply,

    A. "Administer eye drops with two drops in the left eye two times a day."
    B. "Administer eye drops with two drops in the left eye three times a day."
    C. "Administer eye drops with two drops in the right eye three times a day."
    D. "Administer eye drops with two drops in the right eye two times a day."

20. Which of the following is a legal document that must be retained for at least 5 years?

    A. Appointment matrix.
    B. Daily appointment schedule.
    C. Telephone message form.
    D. Diagnostic procedure tracking log.

21. When a patient has two (or more) health plans, the CMAA should initially

    A. determine which plan provides best coverage.
    B. determine which plans provide primary and secondary (tertiary, etc.) coverage.
    C. ask the patient to choose which plan to use.
    D. assume both plans will pay for coverage.

22. "H & P" in a medical record refers to

    A. healthcare provider.
    B. help and provisions.
    C. health priorities.
    D. history and physical.

23. Pre-testing instructions should be provided to the patient

    A. in printed form.
    B. verbally (in person or over the telephone).
    C. verbally (in person or over the telephone) and in printed form.
    D. verbally and in printed form at the request of the patient.

24. if a practice schedules 3 to 4 patients every hour so that they all arrive at the same time and are seen in the order in which they arrive, the type of scheduling utilized is

    A. fixed scheduled appointments.
    B. tidal wave/open hour booking.
    C. clustering.
    D. wave booking.

25. If a practice that carries out HIV/AIDS testing uses an alphanumeric code instead of the patient's name for testing, this code is referred to as a(n)

    A. secret code.
    B. unique identifier.
    C. alternate name.
    D. confidential identifier.

26. Which of the following terms refers to a physician who specializes in care, treatment and surgery of musculoskeletal problems?

    A. Orthopedist.
    B. Radiologist.
    C. Rheumatologist.
    D. Physiatrist.

27. The protective strategy for insurance companies that involves limiting the maximum dollar benefits for a policy is a

    A. reinsurance.
    B. deferred liability.
    C. cap.
    D. third-party liability.

28. If a patient cancels an appointment, this cancellation must be documented in

    A. the appointment matrix.
    B. the appointment matrix, the daily appointment schedule, and the patient's medical record.
    C. the medical record.
    D. the appointment matrix and the patient's medical record.

29. A patient with autism becomes very distressed and disruptive if made to wait for extended times for an appointment but dislikes getting up early in the morning. If appointments are scheduled in 15-minute increments between 8:00 and 4:00 PM with an hour break from noon to 1:00 PM, what is the best time to schedule the patient?

    A. 8:00 AM.
    B. 11:45 AM.
    C. 1:00 PM.
    D. 3:45 PM.

30. A fee schedule generally contains

    A. names of procedures and charges.
    B. names of procedures, charges, and ICD-10-CM codes.
    C. ICD-10-CM codes, CPT codes, names of procedures, and charges.
    D. names of procedures, charges, and CPT codes.

31. When an insurance plan negotiates a specific fee for a procedure (including all charges) and pays one bill, this is referred to as

    A. unbundling.
    B. bundling.
    C. fee-for-service.
    D. discounted fee-for-service.

32. Because a patient has missed two appointments, the physician instructs the CMAA to tell the patient no appointment times are available the next time the patient calls for an appointment. This is an example of

    A. abandonment.
    B. negligence.
    C. termination.
    D. malpractice.

33. The type of managed care plan that allows a patient to see physicians and care providers within a network but to seek outside treatment in some circumstances is
    A. health maintenance organization (HMO).
    B. exclusive provider organization (EPO).
    C. point of service plan (POS).
    D. preferred provider organization (PPO).

34. If appointments must be cancelled because the physician is having surgery for removal of a tumor, patients should be advised that
    A. the physician is having surgery to remove a tumor.
    B. the physician is unavailable.
    C. the physician is ill.
    D. the office must cancel appointments.

35. The Centers for Disease Control and Prevention is commonly referred to as the
    A. CDCP
    B. DCP.
    C. CCP.
    D. CDC.

36. If a physician states that she wants a procedure carried out "STAT," this means
    A. immediately.
    B. after a meal.
    C. as needed.
    D. per injection.

37. The government entity that requires that personal protective equipment be readily available at the worksite and in appropriate sizes is the
    A. CDC.
    B. FDA.
    C. OSHA.
    D. CMS.

38. If a patient needs preauthorization for an MRI, the CMAA should generally
    A. telephone the insurance company and request preauthorization.
    B. fill out the preauthorization form and fax it to the insurance company.
    C. ask the patient to contact the insurance company regarding preauthorization.
    D. ask the physician to call the insurance company for preauthorization.

39. If extended wait times for patients are common in a practice, the best solution is to
    A. review scheduling practices.
    B. work more efficiently.
    C. provide adequate reading material and/or videos in the waiting area.
    D. apologize to those waiting.

40. If a patient calls for a referral appointment on the advice of the patient's primary physician, the first thing the CMAA should do is to

    A. make an appointment for the patient.
    B. ask the patient about the urgency of the appointment.
    C. obtain the patient's medical records.
    D. ask if the physician wants to accept the referral.

41. The acronym HIPAA stands for

    A. Health Insurance Providers Accountability Act.
    B. Health Insurance Portability and Accountability Act.
    C. Health Initiative and Providers Accountability Act.
    D. Health Information and Priorities Accountability Act.

42. The best solution to dealing with a patient who expresses extreme prejudice toward ethnic minorities and gays is to

    A. tell the patient his attitude is reprehensible.
    B. refuse to work with the patient.
    C. provide minimal service and avoid interacting with patient.
    D. provide professional service and avoid arguing.

43. Which of the following terms refers to a legal writ (order) requiring a person to come to court, testify in court, or bring documents to court?

    A. Subpoena.
    B. Deposition.
    C. Affidavit.
    D. Attachment.

44. An appropriate statement for a CMAA to make on a social networking site about working with patients is

    A. "I really like some of my patients, especially the older woman who calls me 'dear.'"
    B. "I had a patient today who threw a screaming fit at me."
    C. no statement whatsoever.
    D. "I have to see way too many patients in a day!"

45. A root that refers to blood is

    A. cephal-
    B. hemat-
    C. arter-
    D. brach-

46. When a patient has signed a release of information form so the healthcare provider can provide information to a therapist, the CMAA should

    A. release all available information.
    B. ask the patient, item by item, what should be released.
    C. release the minimum information necessary to meet the request.
    D. edit the information released to the therapist.

47. The femur is the bone located in the
   A. thigh.
   B. lower leg.
   C. upper arm.
   D. lower arm.

48. Following right hip transplantation, the patient has been told to avoid adduction. This means that the patient should not
   A. cross the ankles.
   B. turn the right foot outward.
   C. sit with knees above the hips.
   D. cross the right leg over the left.

49. Which of the following terms used to describe breath sounds refers to high or low-pitched whistling or musical sounds?
   A. Rales.
   B. Wheezes.
   C. Rhonchi.
   D. Stridor.

50. Which of the following suffixes means "surgical removal?"
   A. -otomy.
   B. -stomy.
   C. -ectomy.
   D. -scopy.

51. Which vaccination is administered to prevent chicken pox in children?
   A. Varicella.
   B. MMR.
   C. HPV.
   D. Herpes zoster.

52. Standard precautions are required for
   A. patients with infectious diseases.
   B. patients with draining wounds.
   C. patients with diarrhea.
   D. all patients.

53. If a patient has wrenched his ankle joint with tearing of the ligaments, this is referred to as a
   A. rupture
   B. strain.
   C. sprain.
   D. dislocation.

54. How many milliliters are in one ounce?
   A. 20.
   B. 30.
   C. 50.
   D. 60.

- 116 -

55. If a CMAA may have occupational exposure to hepatitis B and the vaccination is recommended,

    A. the CMAA must pay for the vaccination.
    B. the vaccination must be provided at no cost.
    C. the CMAA may bill personal insurance for the vaccination.
    D. the vaccination cannot be declined.

56. Which of the following is appropriate in documenting patient care?

    A. Documenting in advance.
    B. Erasing statements made in error.
    C. Using ditto marks to save time.
    D. Writing in black or blue permanent ink.

57. The purpose of the Joint Commission's "Do-Not-Use" List is to

    A. promote standardization in documentation.
    B. prevent errors.
    C. promote cost-effectiveness.
    D. comply with FDA regulations.

58. The information in a patient's medical record legally belongs to

    A. the physician.
    B. the medical practice/facility.
    C. the patient.
    D. the state.

59. The correct term for a rapid heartbeat is

    A. arrhythmia.
    B. dysrhythmia.
    C. bradycardia.
    D. tachycardia.

60. Which of the following is a violation of patient's confidentiality?

    A. Password-protected computerized charting.
    B. Computer screen for electronic charting facing an open hallway.
    C. Providing report to a minor child's parents.
    D. Describing patient's behavior to the patient's attending physician.

61. What does the following symbol mean?

    A. Biohazard.
    B. Poison.
    C. Irritant.
    D. Health hazard.

62. Personal protective equipment includes all of the following EXCEPT

    A. gloves.
    B. face shields.
    C. uniform.
    D. gown.

63. If a female patient's medical history includes "Para 2, gravida 3," this means that the patient has had

    A. 2 stillbirths and 3 deliveries.
    B. 2 normal deliveries and 3 stillbirths.
    C. 3 deliveries and 2 pregnancies.
    D. 2 deliveries and 3 pregnancies.

64. When taking a patient's temperature with an electronic ear (tympanic) thermometer, the temperature usually registers within

    A. 2 seconds.
    B. 10 to 60 seconds.
    C. 1 to 3 minutes.
    D. 3 to 5 minutes.

65. Which section of the abdomen is the epigastric region?

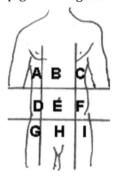

    A. A.
    B. B.
    C. E.
    D. H.

66. If a patient is severely hearing impaired but is able to read lips fairly well and has slight hearing from hearing aids, the CMAA should

    A. speak loudly and stand one to two feet away from the patient.
    B. enunciate very carefully and avoid making distracting gestures.
    C. write out communications on a whiteboard or on the computer for patient to read.
    D. speak slowly and clearly from three to six feet, facing the patient, and use gestures.

67. The correct plural for *vertebra* is

    A. vertebraes.
    B. vertebrae.
    C. vertebras.
    D. vertebrea.

- 118 -

68. When a new patient checks in, the CMAA should confirm identity with

    A. the patient's name and address.
    B. the patients name and birthdate.
    C. two forms of ID with at least one a photo ID.
    D. one form of ID.

69. When scheduling diagnostic procedures for a patient, the CMAA should first

    A. verify that services are covered under the patient's insurance plan.
    B. ask the patient if services are covered under the patient's insurance plan.
    C. inform the patient that the insurance company may not cover costs.
    D. schedule the procedure and advise the patient to check with the insurance.

70. The best method of obtaining copayment from a patient is to state

    A. "Your copayment is $20.00."
    B. "Can you make your $20.00 copayment?"
    C. "I think you have a $20.00 copayment due."
    D. "How would you like to make your $20.00 copayment."

71. If the answering machine shows four patients called requesting visits, which of the following patients should be scheduled first

- T. Stanton: Burning and frequency of urination, low-grade fever.
- S. Locke: Intermittent abdominal cramping and diarrhea X 4 in 12 hours.
- W. Barrett: Flu, cough, increasing shortness of breath.
- E. Nehlich: Persistent short-term memory loss.

    A. T. Stanton.
    B. S. Locke.
    C. W. Barrett.
    D. E. Nehlich.

72. If a patient responds to the CMAA slowly and in very broken English, the CMAA should

    A. ask for a translator before proceeding.
    B. speak slowly and loudly to make sure the patient understands.
    C. rely on pictures and sign language to communicate meaning.
    D. ask what language the patient speaks at home and if the patient can understand.

73. If a patient by the name of Jennifer Brown presents an insurance card with the name of Mary Jones at a visit, the most likely reason is

```
┌─────────────────────────────────────┐
│ Model Insurance                      │
│ Subscriber: Mary Jones               │
│ ID #: ICU44444222286F                │
│ Group #: 777888226DM                 │
│ Plan Code: 066                       │
│                                      │
│ Office visit copay: $25.00           │
│ ER copay: $100.00                    │
│                                      │
│ Verify ID.                    PPO    │
└─────────────────────────────────────┘
```

   A. the patient stole the insurance card from Mary Jones.
   B. the patient is covered under Mary Jones' family plan.
   C. the patient is attempting to use a friend's card.
   D. the patient accidentally brought the wrong card.

74. If paper health records are filed using terminal digit filing and a patient's health record is numbered 44-62-10, in which section will the chart be filed?

   A. Section 44.
   B. Section 62.
   C. Section 10.
   D. Either Section 10 or section 44.

75. If a patient is part of an HMO and needs a regular referral (non-emergent) to see a specialist, gaining approval usually takes

   A. 24 hours.
   B. 2 to 3 days.
   C. 3 to 10 days.
   D. 2 to 3 weeks.

76. If, in the waiting area where other patients are present, the CMAA asks a patient the reason for his visit, this is an example of

   A. a fact finding.
   B. carelessness.
   C. a screening question.
   D. a HIPAA violation.

77. The purpose of an Advance Beneficiary Notice is to

   A. make decisions about end-of-life care.
   B. notify patients that they have been overcharged for a service.
   C. notify patients that services are covered by Medicare.
   D. notify patients that a service may not be covered by Medicare.

78. If a patient's record indicates that the patient has developed folate (vitamin B-12) deficiency anemia because of long-term use of the drug metformin for diabetic treatment, which ICD-10-CM diagnostic code is appropriate?

    A. D52.0 Dietary folate deficiency anemia.
    B. D52.1 Drug-induced folate deficiency anemia.
    C. D52.8 Other folate deficiency anemias.
    D. D52.9 Folate deficiency anemia, unspecified.

79. The *guarantor* of an account is the

    A. insurance company that will provide payment for claims.
    B. the person for whom the account is established.
    C. the person who is responsible for paying bills not paid for by insurance.
    D. the person show is responsible for signing consent forms.

80. When setting up user accounts, which of the following would be classified as a strong password?

    A. Carolina.
    B. Ilovemycat.
    C. 12161980
    D. D36&lobx.

81. Where in the patient's record would the following list be found?

    • Ambulatory as desired.
    • Acetaminophen 100 mg every 6 hours prn pain.
    • Bactrim DS 800/160 mg twice daily for 6 days.

    A. Physician's orders.
    B. Nursing notes.
    C. Physician's progress notes.
    D. Medication record.

82. In terms of filing claims, "bundling" refers to

    A. sending a number of different claims at the same time.
    B. including a number of different procedures under one code.
    C. separating linked procedures into different codes.
    D. including both CPT codes and ICD-10-PCS codes on claims.

83. If a patient tells the CMAA that the physician has recommended the patient see a podiatrist (foot specialist) for nail care and asks whom to see, the CMAA should

    A. refer to the practice's list of recommended referrals.
    B. suggest one or two names with whom the CMAA is familiar.
    C. decline to provide any information.
    D. tell the patient to check in a physician's directory.

84. Which of the following allows the designated person to make all legal decisions for a patient, including decisions about health care, even if the patient remains competent?

    A. Living will.
    B. Advance directive.
    C. Health care proxy.
    D. Durable power of attorney.

85. According to the following accounts aging report, how many accounts are delinquent?

#	Name	Filed	Amount	Current	31-60	61-90	91-120	120+	Balance total
1	T. Jones	2-10-19	$200.00	$200.00					$200.00
2	R. Moore	1-4-19	$100.00		$100				$100.00
3	M. Show	12-3-18	$480.00			$480.00			$480.00

    A. None.
    B. One.
    C. Two.
    D. Three.

86. In a tickler file, a copy of a submitted claim is generally placed under the day that is
    A. 2 weeks after the submission date.
    B. 3 weeks after the submission date.
    C. 4 weeks after the submission date.
    D. 6 weeks after the submission date.

87. A pre-invoice is used to
    A. bill for services.
    B. provide an estimate of costs of services.
    C. prepare an invoice.
    D. estimate discounts to apply to the invoice.

88. Which of the following is an example of correct ergonomics?
    A. Hold weight close to the body instead of at arm's length.
    B. Pull instead of pushing, rolling, or sliding.
    C. Flex at the waist to pick up an item.
    D. Reach overhead for no more than 30 inches.

89. When screening a patient over the telephone, it is essential that the CMAA
    A. refer the call to a nurse.
    B. ask questions as seems appropriate.
    C. ask everyone the same questions.
    D. follow a screening manual.

90. If a CMAA receives a needlestick injury from a needle and syringe inadvertently thrown into the trash, the first step should be to
    A. log the injury in the needlestick and sharps log.
    B. report the injury to a supervisor.
    C. thoroughly wash the area with soap and water.
    D. ask for an HIV test and prophylaxis.

91. If a physician bills for a service at a higher level than that actually provided, this is an example of
    A. switching.
    B. upcoding.
    C. downcoding.
    D. doubling.

92. If a chemical spills in the office, before cleaning up the spill, the CMAA should immediately
 A. consult the Safety Data Sheet (SDS).
 B. call the poison center for instructions.
 C. pour a neutralizing substance on the spill.
 D. wear a gas mask and personal protective equipment.

93. If a physician routinely bills for a comprehensive exam for all Medicare patients, regardless of their symptoms or complaints, this is an example of
 A. Medicare fraud.
 B. legal practice.
 C. medical malpractice.
 D. standard procedure.

94. OSHA's general duty clause states that
 A. an emergency evacuation plan must be in place.
 B. personal protective equipment must be provided.
 C. the workplace must be free of hazards that may result in harm.
 D. employment training must be documented.

95. If the physician has ordered that a patient enter an alcohol rehabilitation program, but the patient refuses to do so, the patient is
 A. violating the physician-patient agreement.
 B. behaving in an inappropriate manner.
 C. acting in an illegal manner.
 D. exercising the right to refuse treatment.

96. When a patient makes an appointment to see a physician and allows the CMAA to take vital signs without expressly giving permission, this is an example of
 A. informed consent.
 B. implied consent.
 C. routine consent.
 D. inadvertent consent.

97. If a staff member takes $20 from petty cash to buy coffee and tea for the breakroom, the CMAA should
 A. put a note in the petty cash box indicating cash was withdrawn.
 B. ask the bookkeeper or accountant to replenish petty cash.
 C. log it into the petty cash record and give the staff member a petty cash receipt.
 D. take no particular action as this is what petty cash is intended for.

98. If a physician refuses to treat a patient with severe disabilities because of the inconvenience caused by needing to use special lifts and equipment, the physician is in violation of
 A. ADA.
 B. OSHA.
 C. HIPAA.
 D. FDA.

- 123 -

99. If a nurse claims to have forgotten his/her password and asks to use the CMAA's password to access a patient's electronic health record, the CMAA should

    A. allow the nurse to use the password.
    B. ask the supervisor if it is all right to share the password.
    C. access the EHR for the nurse.
    D. refuse to allow the nurse to use the password.

100. Which of the following is a combined federal and state welfare program to assist people with low incomes with payment for medical care?

    A. Medicare.
    B. Medicaid.
    C. SafetyNet.
    D. Tricare.

101. Which of the following medical claim forms is used by physicians and out-patient medical practices?

    A. CMS 1557.
    B. CMS 1554.
    C. CMS 1500.
    D. CMS 1450.

102. Is the following sign-in sheet HIPAA compliant?

Sign-in sheet: June 15						
#	Full name	Birthdate	Arrival time	Appt. time	Physician	New (√)
1	Sarah J. Jacobs	5-13-80	8:00	15	Jones	
2	Brad Lincoln	2-10-65	8:25	8:30	Jones	√

    A. Yes, it is HIPAA compliant.
    B. No, it should not include the birthdate.
    C. No, it should not include the birthdate or full name.
    D. No, it should not include the full name or new patient indication.

103. A necessary component of informed consent prior to a procedure is

    A. Names of assisting staff members.
    B. Beginning and ending times.
    C. Risks and benefits of procedure.
    D. Facility statistics regarding procedure.

104. Medicare recipients are required to pay a certain amount out-of-pocket each year before Medicare starts paying. This is a

    A. deductible.
    B. co-insurance.
    C. copayment.
    D. cap.

105. The dollar amount that an insurance company considers payment in full for a claim is the

   A. cap.
   B. full amount.
   C. allowed amount.
   D. contingency fee.

106. If a CMAA must create a number of different documents (letters, calendar, fax cover sheet) in a word processing program, the first step should be to

   A. ask others for advice.
   B. search for templates.
   C. sketch out possible formats.
   D. gather samples.

107. If first-class postage for an envelope weighing up to one ounce is $0.55, how much postage is required for an envelope weighing 1.5 ounces?

   A. $0.70.
   B. $0.83.
   C. $1.00.
   D. $1.10.

108. If a medical practice uses electronic health records and has an image-based backup system for both local and distant backup, how often should backups of data be done?

   A. Every hour.
   B. Every 8 hours.
   C. Every 24 hours.
   D. Every week.

109. If a CMAA is faxing sensitive information about a patient to another healthcare provider, the most important action for the CMAA is to

   A. call to ensure the fax went through.
   B. mark the fax as "confidential."
   C. call ahead to say the fax is coming.
   D. deidentify the material.

110. If a CMAA sees that another staff member has posted a picture of a patient on Facebook with negative comments about the patient's weight and mental health issues, the CMAA should immediately

   A. tell the staff member to remove the picture and comments.
   B. report the matter to a supervisor at work.
   C. report the matter to HIPAA.
   D. ignore the matter since access to the page is limited to friends.

111. If the front desk is sometimes left unattended when patients arrive, the best solution is likely to

   A. play a prerecorded greeting every few minutes.
   B. notify patients when they schedule their appointments.
   C. assume patients will understand what to do.
   D. post a sign asking patients to sign in and take a seat.

112. The purpose of a firewall is to

A. prevent fire from spreading.
B. block unauthorized access to computer programs.
C. encrypt data being transmitted.
D. protect information left on the monitor.

113. If a new patient is scheduled two weeks in the future, the CMAA should

A. telephone and go over the demographic form with the patient.
B. mail the demographic form to the patient to fill out before the visit.
C. take no further action until the patient actually arrives.
D. advise the patient that he can download the demographic form.

114. If the CMAA is typing a letter in MS Word and accidentally deletes a paragraph, the CMAA should

A. retype the paragraph.
B. run an application to retrieve data.
C. select the "undo typing" command or button.
D. select the "find" command and enter key words.

115. The primary advantage of just-in-time ordering of inventory is

A. time saving.
B. cost saving.
C. flexibility.
D. labor saving.

116. Which of the following types of negligence refers to willfully providing inadequate care without regard to the safety and security of the client?

A. Contributory negligence.
B. Comparative negligence.
C. Negligent conduct.
D. Gross negligence.

117. A patient with a history of mental disease begins swearing and pacing back and forth in the waiting area, shouting, "You can't make me stay here!" The most appropriate initial response is to

A. speak calmly and quietly to the client.
B. tell the client this behavior is inappropriate.
C. leave the room.
D. call security to restrain the client.

118. When entering the room of a patient who is deaf and facing away from the door, the CMAA should

A. approach from the direction the client is facing.
B. say the client's name.
C. approach and touch the client.
D. clap hands or tap the foot.

119. When the physician is almost ready to see a patient, the CMAA should generally place the patient's medical record

    A. in the examining room.
    B. in the physician's hand.
    C. in the file holder, name facing inward.
    D. In the file holder, name facing outward.

120. When using a computer, the monitor should be adjusted so that the user's eyes are in a line that is

    A. at the top of the monitor casing.
    B. 2 to 3 inches below the top of the monitor casing.
    C. 3-5 inches below the top of the monitor casing.
    D. 1 to 2 inches above the bottom of the monitor casing.

121. Which of the following is a nonverbal clue that a patient may be anxious?

    A. Patient rubs his eyes and yawns.
    B. Patient concentrates of cell phone and sends text messages.
    C. Patient's pupils are constricted and patient sniffs repeatedly.
    D. Patient rubs hands together constantly.

122. When a patient's spouse asks for information about another patient, the response that complies with the Health Insurance Portability and Accountability Act (HIPAA) is

    A. "The law doesn't allow me to give out any information about patients in order to protect their privacy and safety."
    B. "His wife is in the waiting area. You can ask her."
    C. "Why are you asking?"
    D. "He has leukemia, like your husband."

123. In MS Excel, which function would be best for adding up all the values in a column?

    A. COUNTA.
    B. ADD.
    C. SUM.
    D. MAX.

124. If the CMAA is using the PASS acronym to guide use of a fire extinguisher, the letters stand for

    A. place, apply, shake, spray.
    B. pick up, adjust, spray, scatter.
    C. prepare, activate, select, spray.
    D. pull, aim, squeeze, spray.

125. When closing the office at the end of the day, the first task should be to

    A. make sure that all staff, visitors, and patients have gone.
    B. turn off all equipment.
    C. notify the answering service or turn on the answering machine.
    D. backup all data.

126. When writing a letter on paper with a letterhead, on which line is the date placed?

A. 1 line below the letterhead.
B. 2 lines below the letterhead.
C. 3 lines below the letterhead.
D. 4 lines below the letterhead.

127. If the CMAA is sending a letter to a patient and wants it delivered within 5 days and wants the receiver to sign for the letter and wants a return receipt, the letter should be sent by

A. registered mail.
B. priority mail.
C. first class mail.
D. certified mail.

128. Purging of files refers to

A. moving a file from active to inactive.
B. moving a file from paper to electronic.
C. removal all unofficial documents from the file.
D. making sure all records are in order.

129. Which of the following terminologies is used to code for medical procedures and services under health insurance plans (both public and private)?

A. CPT.
B. ICD-10-CM.
C. NOC.
D. NIC.

130. What is the correct alphabetical order for the following files (first to last)?

- Sam C. Smith.
- S. C. Smith
- Sarah St. John.
- Trudy Santa Maria.
- Dana Snyder.
- Jacob Smithson.

A. Sarah St. John, Trudy Santa Maria, Sam C. Smith, S.C. Smith, Jacob Smithson, and Dana Snyder.
B. Sarah Saint John, Trudy Santa Maria, Jacob Smithson, S.C. Smith, Sam C. Smith, and Dana Synder.
C. Trudy Santa Maria, Jacob Smithson, S.C. Smith, Sam C. Smith, Dana Snyder, and Sarah St. John.
D. Trudy Santa Maria, S.C. Smith, Sam C. Smith, Jacob Smithson, Dana Synder, and Sarah St. John.

Answer Key and Explanations

1. B: If, while answering service takes calls during the night, numerous patients have complained that telephone calls during working hours are often unanswered, the best solution for the office is likely to ask the answering service to answer calls after a specified number of rings (usually 3 to 4). If an office has limited staff, the person who answers the call may need to assist the physician or may be on another line and unable to take a call.

2. D: If a patient in the waiting room is coughing, the CMAA should provide the patient with a face mask, explaining that the office policy is to ask all patients with a cough to wear one to prevent spread of infection. Droplets from cough can remain suspended for up to 10 minutes in the air. The patient should be moved to an examining room as soon as one is available to reduce the risk of exposure to others but should not be asked to wait outside.

3. A: OSHA's **form 301** is used to describe each workplace death/injury (what actually happened) in detail, including the date and time, the type of injury, the cause, the individuals involved, and a description of what the person was doing immediately before the incident. This form must be submitted to OSHA with one week of being notified of the death/injury. **Form 300** is a log used to list each workplace death/injury that occurs at a workplace. Form **300A** is an annual summary of all workplace deaths/injuries that have occurred.

4. B: An example of protected health information includes a patient's diagnosis and any information regarding the patient's health condition or treatment, any identifying information, and any information regarding payment for healthcare that can identify the patient. The sexual abuse of a child must be reported to the appropriate authorities, such as Child Protective Services. Information that is shared, such as for research, must first be de-identified so that the information cannot be traced back to specific individuals.

5. C: If the physician has indicated on the patient's encounter form that the patient should return for a follow-up exam in one week but there are no appointment times available for one month, the CMA should ask the physician if the patient can wait one month. If not, then the patient should be double-booked but informed there might be a short wait at the visit. If a cancellation occurs, the patient can be rescheduled.

6. A: A commonly-used analgesic is acetaminophen (Tylenol). Analgesics are medications used to control pain and may include over-the-counter drugs, such as acetaminophen and ibuprofen, and prescription drugs, such as codeine and morphine. Acetaminophen is often advised for mild to moderate pain and to control fever. It is generally a safe drug for both children and adults if dosage recommendations are followed. An overdose of acetaminophen can result in damage to the liver.

7. D: The distal part of the arm is the part near the wrist and hand. Distal refers to furthest from the point of reference. With limbs, the distal part is toward the hand and foot and the proximal, which is closest to the point of reference, is toward the shoulder and hip. *Proximal* and *distal* are terms often used to describe the location of an injury or abnormality.

8. C: When using a copier or scanner for medical records, it is essential to remove stored information from memory to prevent unauthorized access. Most current equipment stores copies of documents scanned or copied. Records should never be left in a basket near the equipment for later scanning or copying. If possible, the equipment should require a password as this helps to trace use and determine who was copying or scanning and when.

9. B: If a new patient calls for an appointment and states that she has been experiencing heavier than usual periods with cramping for the past 3 months, the type of appointment would be categorized as new, non-urgent problem/illness. Since this is an ongoing problem and the patient is unlikely at risk if the appointment is delayed, the patient can wait for an appointment time if necessary although the patient should be scheduled as soon as possible because "heavy period" can have different meanings to different people.

10. A: **Beneficence** is the principle that requires that actions should be carried out for the good (benefit) of the patient. **Maleficence** is the principle that requires that care should be provided in such a way as to avoid intentional harm. **Justice** requires that limited healthcare benefits be distributed fairly. **Autonomy** refers to the right that the individual has to make decisions about his or her own care, including the right to consent and to refuse care.

11. D: If three patients cancel appointments for the same morning, the best solution is to call those on the list for wanting an earlier appointment and to reschedule three of them for the empty time periods. Most busy practices have patients who wanted earlier appointments but no earlier time periods were available at that time, so practices should keep a list of these patients and contact them when cancellations occur because cancelled result in wasted time and less income.

12. C: **Indemnity insurance** pays in the form of predetermined payments for loss or damages rather than for healthcare service. **Liability insurance** pays damages for bodily injury or loss of property, such as from injury resulting from unsafe conditions. **No-fault auto insurance** pays for injury/damages resulting from driving a car with coverage varying according to state regulations. **Accident and health insurance** pays for healthcare costs and may or may not include disability payments, depending on the type of policy.

13. A: The vertical plane that separates anterior (front) from posterior (back) is the coronal/frontal plane.

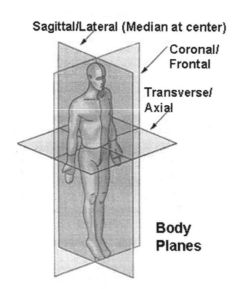

14. D: If a new patient being scheduled is complaining of increasing edema (swelling) of the feet and shortness of breath, then the patient should be scheduled for longer than 10 minutes because the physician will need time to take a history and physical and to examine the patient to determine the likely diagnosis and best course of treatment. The first longer time period available begins at 9:00

- 130 -

AM on June 6. Because the patient is complaining of shortness of breath, the appointment should not be delayed until June 7.

15. B: If a physician informs the CMAA that she would like to have a conference call with three other physicians at 8:30 AM on the following Monday, the first thing the CMAA should do is to contact all participants to verify the correct telephone numbers, the data, and time to ensure that the others will be available and expecting the call. The CMAA should be sure to block out the time on the appointment matrix so that no patients are scheduled for the physician during the call.

16. C: The percentage of costs that a patient must pay is the **co-insurance**. For example, if the insurance company pays 80%, then the co-insurance is 20%. In some cases, such as Medicare, the patient may carry a supplementary/secondary insurance that covers the co-insurance amount although the patient may still be required to pay a **deductible** (a dollar amount rather than a percentage amount). **Cap** refers to the maximum amount that an insurance carrier will pay. **Co-payment** is the specific dollar amount required for each visit or service.

17. C: The most effective method of decreasing no shows is to remind the patients of appointments a day or two before. Studies show giving reminders (usually by telephone or text message) often reduces the number of no shows by half. If, however, some patients still are no shows, many practices charge a set fee, such as $25 for a missed visit, but patients must be notified in advance (generally at the time the appointment is made) that a fee is charged for missed appointments.

18. A: **Subjective** notes usually quote what the client states directly:" I think this is a waste of time!" **Objective** notes record what is observed, clinical facts: "Patient sitting with face flushed." **Assessment** relates to evaluation of subjective and objective notes: "Patient appears anxious and complains of being very busy at work. BP 132.86, P. 18." **Plan** is based on assessment: "Review medication list and instruct patient in self-monitoring of blood pressure."

19. C: If the physician has given the patient directions that state "Eye drops--gtt ii OD TID" and the patient asks what it means, the CMAA would reply: ""Administer eye drops with two drops in the right eye three times a day." Roman numerals are often used in medical prescriptions, but sometimes in lower case—ii instead of II—because the dots help to reinforce the number.

Roman numerals (often used in prescriptions)	I = 1, V = 5, X = 10, L = 50, C = 100, D = 500, and M = 1000	IV = 4, V = 5, VII = 7, IX =9, XII = 12 XLII = 42

20. B: The daily appointment schedule is a legal document that must be retained for at least 5 years. The daily appointment schedule is a list of patients who are to be seen that day including contact information (telephone number) and the purpose of the visit. If created in a word processing program, it should be printed and any additions, deletions, or corrections made in permanent ink. The appointment schedule is used to pull medical records if the practice utilizes paper records or to access electronic records.

21. B: When patients have two or more health plans, the CMAA should initially determine which plan provides primary coverage and which secondary coverage and so on. Rules vary widely regarding the order of payment, so the CMAA may need to contact the health plans and determine the order of insurance responsibility on an individual basis. Double coverage is usually precluded, and the patient is often not able to choose. Medicare is primary over supplementary insurances, and private insurances are primary over Medicaid.

22. D. "H & P" in the medical record refers to history and physical. Other commonly used abbreviations include:

- Hx = history.
- Dx = diagnosis.
- Tx = Treatment
- I & O = intake and output.
- DOI = date of injury.
- DOB = date of birth.
- AMA = against medical advice.
- NKA = no known allergies.

23. C: Pre-testing instructions should be provided to the patient verbally in person or over the telephone and in printed form (paper or electronic). The CMAA must not assume that patients can read and understand printed instructions or will take the time to do so, but should always review instructions verbally with a patient and ask for feedback to ensure the patient understands. The instructions (verbal and printed) should be noted in the patient's medical record.

24. D: **Wave booking** occurs if a practice schedules 3 to 4 patients every hour so that they all arrive at the same time and are seen in the order in which they arrive. With **fixed scheduled appointments**, each patient is generally scheduled to see the health provider at a specific time, such as at 9 AM, and no other patient is scheduled at the same time. With **tidal wave/open hour booking**, anyone can come during a specified time period and be seen on a first-come, first-served basis or according to acuity. With **clustering**, only one type of patient or those having similar procedures are scheduled during a block of time.

25. B: If a practice that carries out HIV/AIDS testing uses an alphanumeric code instead of the patient's name for testing, this code is referred to as a unique identifier because each patient is given a different code and uses that rather than the patient's name. Unique identifiers are often used to encourage members of key populations, such as sex-workers and drug abusers, to have testing when their concerns about confidentiality may otherwise prevent them from doing so.

26. A: **Orthopedist** refers to a physician who specializes in care, treatment and surgery of musculoskeletal problems, such as bone fractures and skeletal abnormalities. A **radiologist** is a physician who specializes in imaging, such as x-rays, CTs, and MRIs, used to detect diseases and abnormalities. A **rheumatologist** is a physician who specializes in the care and treatment of those with rheumatic diseases or conditions with generalized inflammation and pain and stiffness of muscles and joints. A **physiatrist** is a physician who specialized in physical medicine and rehabilitation.

27. C: The protective strategy for insurance companies that involves limiting the maximum dollar benefits for a policy is a cap. Caps may vary depending on the type of insurance. A routine accident and health benefits plan for one person may set a specific dollar maximum for that person, but a family plan may set a plan cap for the entire family and individual caps. Automobile insurance that covers bodily injury also usually has a category cap (such as $1 million for bodily injury) and per person caps (such as $250,000 per person), so one injured person cannot receive the entire amount.

28. B: If a patient cancels an appointment, it should be noted in the appointment matrix and the daily appointment record by crossing the appointment time out in red and writing "cancelled" or "C" and signing. The cancellation should also be reported in the patient's medical record along with

the reason if known. This is especially important if the patient develops complications because of the missed appointment. However, if the patient simply reschedules, this information does not need to be noted in the medical record.

29. C: The two best times to schedule a patient to avoid extended wait times is the first appointment of the day (8:00 AM) and first appointment after lunch (1:00 PM). Because this patient does not like to get up early in the morning, the early AM appointment should be avoided and the patient scheduled for 1:00 PM. If wait time is inevitable, the patient may cope better if placed in an examining room rather than left in the waiting area.

30. D: A fee schedule should contain a list of procedures, the providers charges, and the appropriate CPT codes. The fee schedule should mirror the charges listed on the encounter form. A practice may, in fact, collect different fees depending on the insurance carrier. Medicare, for example, may only pay a percentage of the fee and many insurance companies negotiate discounts. This means that, effectively, a practice may have many actual fee schedules when discounts and contractual agreements are considered.

31. B: **Bundling** occurs when an insurance plan negotiates a specific fee for a procedure, including all associated costs, and pays one bill. **Unbundling** occurs when a bundled agreement is dissolved, and the insurance plan pays separate bills (hospital, anesthesiologist, surgeon, etc.). **Fee-for-service** is the traditional billing method in which services are billed for separately. **Discounted fee-for-service** is similar to fee-for-service except that reimbursements are discounted.

32. A: If, because a patient has missed two appointments, the physician instructs the CMAA to tell the patient no appointment times are available the next time the patient calls for an appointment, this is an example of abandonment. If a patient is to be terminated from a practice, the patient must be sent written notice explaining the reason and allowing the patient to make other arrangements for care.

33. C: A point of service plan (POS) is a structure that combines aspects of an HMO with a PPO. Patients are able to receive care from healthcare providers within the network or may seek treatment outside the network in some circumstances. This type of plan offers more flexibility to the patient, but usually there are additional costs when a patient chooses to seek treatment outside of the network. Co-payments may increase and the percentage of costs covered by the plan may decrease.

34. B: If appointments must be cancelled because the physician is having surgery for removal of a tumor, patients should be advised that the physician is unavailable. Giving no reason is frustrating to patients, but giving details about the physician's illness, or even the fact that the physician is ill, is a violation of the physician's right to privacy under HIPAA regulations. If patients have acute problems or the physician will be unavailable for a prolonged period, then recommendations for obtaining medical care elsewhere should be provided.

35. D: The Centers for Disease Control and Prevention, a federal agency under the Department of Health and Human Services, is commonly referred to as the CDC. The CDC leads the government efforts at prevention of illness and health promotion. The CDC collects data regarding infectious diseases and investigates and helps to develop methods to control outbreaks and promote public health. The CDC provides information about infectious disease for the public and for healthcare practitioners.

36. A: If a physician states that she wants a procedure carried out "stat," this mean immediately. For example, the physician may want diagnostic tests to be carried out stat or medications administered stat. Other commonly-used abbreviations include:

- prn = as needed
- ac = before meals
- pc =after meals
- PO = by mouth
- ASAP = as soon as possible.

37. C: The government entity that requires that personal protective equipment be readily available at the worksite and in appropriate sizes is the Occupational Safety and Health Administration (OSHA). OSHA sets and enforces regulations related to workplace safety. In healthcare, this encompasses bloodborne pathogens, hazardous materials and hazardous wastes, and compressed gases and air equipment. OSHA also establishes lifting limits and ergonomic guidelines to minimize the risk of injury. Compliance officers can take complaints and issue citations for those out of compliance.

38. B: If a patient needs preauthorization for an MRI, the CMAA should generally fill out the preauthorization form and fax it to the insurance company. This is more efficient than telephoning because the insurance company needs the information on the form, which usually contains the patient's name and demographic information, information about the healthcare provider, patient preliminary diagnosis and diagnostic code, information about the insurance plan, planned procedure and appropriate codes, amount of patient's copayment and/or deductible, hospital benefits, and contact information.

39. A: If extended wait times for patients are common in a practice, the best solution is to review scheduling practices to try to identify and remedy the cause. For example, some free time may be left in the schedule, or patients scheduled for longer appointment times. In all cases of wait times for more than 10 to 15 minutes, the CMAA should acknowledge the wait time, apologize, estimate the additional wait time, provide comfort measures, and offer options, such as rescheduling.

40. C: If a patient calls for a referral on the advice of the patient's primary physician, the first thing the CMAA should do it so obtain medical records so that the physician can review the records and determine the urgency. Then, the CMAA should call the patient and set up an appointment. If time permits, the CMAA may send medical history forms to the patient to fill out prior to the visit or may ask the patient to come to the appointment 15 minutes early in order to fill out the forms.

41. B: The acronym HIPAA stands for Health Insurance Portability and Accountability Act. HIPAA addresses the rights of individual related to privacy and confidentiality of health information. Healthcare providers must not release any information or documentation about a patient's condition or treatment without consent, as the individual has the right to determine who has access to personal information. Personal information about the patient is considered protected health information (PHI), and consists of any identifying or personal information about the patient, such as health history, condition, or treatments in any form, and any documentation, including electronic, verbal, or written.

42. D: The best solution to dealing with a patient who expresses extreme prejudice toward ethnic minorities and gays is to provide professional services and avoid arguing. The CMAA should stay focused on the needs of the patient rather than the patient's attitudes. CMAAs often encounter

ethical conflicts and patients with value systems at odds with their own, and trying to change the patients' ideas is generally ineffective and just leads to conflict.

43. A: A **subpoena** is a legal writ (order) that requires a person to come to court, testify in court, and/or produce documents. A **deposition** is testimony that a person gives under oath in response to questions, usually in a lawyer's office rather than in a court. An **affidavit** is a written statement provided under oath. An **attachment** is a lien on property/assets (such as a bank account) to pay for money owed.

44. C: An appropriate statement for a CMAA to make on a social networking site about working with patients is no statement whatsoever! The CMAA should not describe patients even in general terms without naming them because people may be able to determine whom the CMAA is referring to by the description. Additionally, complaining about work ("I have to see way too many patients...") suggests that the CMAA is not able to give adequate attention to patients.

45. B: A root that refers to blood is *hemat-*, such as in hematology and hematocrit. Another root that refers to blood is *sanguin-,* such as in sanguinous (bloody). The root *cephal-* refers to the head, such as in cephalic while *encephal-* refers to the brain (in the head), such as in encephalitis. *Arter-* or *arteri-* refers to arteries, such as in arteriogram (picture of arteries). *Brach-* refers to the arm, such as the brachial artery (located in the arm).

46. C: When a patient has signed a release of information form so the healthcare provider can provide information to a therapist or any other individual, the CMAA should release the minimum information necessary to meet the request. If for example, the request does not include the dates prior to a current injury, then the CMAA should not include those with the records released. Even when records are released, the CMAA should remain aware of the patient's right to confidentiality and privacy.

47. A: The femur is the bone located in the thigh.

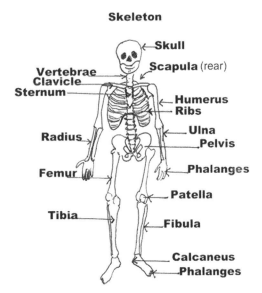

Skeleton

48. D: Following hip transplantation, residents are routinely advised to avoid adduction (movement toward the body or across midline) to prevent dislocation of the prosthesis. This means that the resident with a right hip transplantation should not cross the right leg over the left but should keep

- 135 -

the legs apart. Adduction is the opposite of abduction, which means to move away from the body. Thus, a patient who avoids adduction is often advised to maintain abduction, keeping the legs apart.

49. B: When describing breath sounds, **wheezes** refer to high or low-pitched whistling or musical sounds. **Rales** are high-pitched crackles usually heard at end of expiration in lung bases indicating fluid in the alveoli (air sacs) and may be fine or coarse. **Rhonchi** are deep rumbling sounds that may be high-pitched and sibilant (whistling) or low-pitched and sonorous (snoring) caused by constricted airways or large amounts of secretions in airways. **Stridor** is the crowing sound caused by inflammation and swelling or larynx and trachea.

50. C: The suffices that means "surgical removal" is -*ectomy.* Common suffixes that refer to procedures include:

-otomy	Incision	Colectomy (incision of the colon)
-ectomy	Surgical removal	Colectomy (surgical removal of the colon), tonsillectomy (surgical removal of the tonsils)
-stomy	Surgical creation of body opening	Colostomy (creation of an opening into the colon), tracheostomy (creation of an opening into the trachea)
-scopy	Examination with a scope	Bronchoscopy (examination of the bronchi with a scope)

51. A: **Varicella** is the vaccination administered to prevent chicken pox in children. **MMR** is administered to prevent measles, mumps, and rubella (German measles). **HPV** is administered to prevent human papillomavirus, which is associated with cancer of the reproductive system. **Herpes zoster** (Shingrix) is used to prevent shingles, which may occur in those who have previously been infected with chickenpox.

25. D: Standard precautions must be used for all patients. Standard precautions include maintaining hand hygiene by using an alcohol-based hand rub or handwashing with soap and water (required for any residue on hands) before touching a patient, when completing care, after any contact with body fluids, and before applying and after removing gloves. Required personal protective equipment includes gloves for contact with body fluids and gowns, facemasks, and goggles or face shields if needed. Standard precautions also include respiratory hygiene and cough etiquette.

53. C: If a patient has wrenched his ankle with tearing of the ligaments, this is referred to as a sprain. Other terms commonly used to describe orthopedic injuries include:

Dislocation	Displacement of a part (generally a bone from a socket), such as a dislocation of the elbow or shoulder.
Fracture	Break in a part, primarily a bone or tooth.
Rupture	Tear and separation, such as a ruptured Achille's tendon.
Strain	Overstretched or torn muscle, such as a hamstring strain.

54. A: One ounce contains 30 milliliters (mL). Medical measurements usually use mL instead of ounce because the metric system can measure smaller quantities more accurately. Common measurements include:

- 4 ounces = 120 mL.
- One cup/8 ounces = 240 mL.
- One pint (16 ounces) = 473 mL (approximately 0.5 liter/500 mL)
- One quart (32 ounces) = 946 mL (approximate 1 liter/1000 mL).

55. B: If a CMAA may have occupational exposure to hepatitis B and the hepatitis B vaccination series is recommended, the vaccination series must be provided at no cost to the CMAA within 10 days of hire, and the practice may not bill the vaccination to the CMAA's insurance. As with all treatment, the CMAA may decline the vaccinations but must sign the declination form to free the practice from liability.

56. D: In documenting patient care, the CMAA should write in blue or black permanent ink only. The CMAA should never document in advance of carrying out a procedure, erase anything on the patient record, or use ditto marks to save time. Documentation should be accurate, written clearly in permanent ink or typed, and done in a timely manner. The CMAA should make sure that the patient's name is present on each page and should leave no blank lines.

57. B: The purpose of the Joint Commission's "Do-Not-Use" List is to prevent errors and protect patient safety by eliminating abbreviations, acronyms, and symbols that can be easily mistaken or misconstrued. In many cases, abbreviations have been eliminated in favor of words (QD is replaced with daily and QID with 4 times daily). With numbers, trailing zeroes are eliminated (7.0 mg is replaced with 7 mg) although leading zero (.7 mg replaced with 0.7 mg) is required. Many symbols (@, <, >.μg) are replaced with words. Acronyms (SOB) are replaced with words. However, some healthcare practitioners persist is using these abbreviations, acronyms, and symbols.

58. C: The information in a patient's medical record legally belongs to the patient, according to the rules of HIPAA; however, the record itself belongs to the physician and organization responsible for its creation. The patient, therefore, has a right to receive copies of any part of the medical record but not the record itself, which must be stored. Holders of the patient's medical record have up to 30 days to comply with a request for records and can apply for an additional 30-day extension. Some state laws have a shorter timetable that applies, so the CMAA should review state requirements.

59. D: **Tachycardia** is the correct term for a rapid heartbeat (over 100 beats per minute in adults). **Bradycardia** means a slow heartbeat (less than 60 beats per minute in adults). The terms dysrhythmia and arrhythmia are used interchangeably to mean an abnormal heartbeat, such as an irregular pulse. The term **fibrillation** is used to describe a rapid, quivering and often irregular ineffectual heartbeat. **Asystole** refers to a cardiac arrest in which there is no heartbeat.

60. B: Charting electronically with a computer screen open to view is a violation of patient's confidentiality because unauthorized personnel and visitors may be able to read the records. Computerized record keeping should always be password protected. Parents have a legal right to information about their minor child unless their child is legally emancipated. Patients have a right to expect that when they divulge personal information to a CMAA that only those with a need to know (such as the physician) will be provided this information.

61. A:

Sign/Symbol	Interpretation
	Biohazard: Includes biological substances, such as body fluids, that pose a threat to humans. Appears on sharps containers that hold contaminated needles.
	Poison: Includes materials, gases, or substances that are extremely toxic and may result in death or severe illness.

	Irritant: Includes material, gases, or substances that are irritants to skin, eyes, and/or respiratory tract, acutely toxic, or have a narcotic effect.
	Health hazard: Includes carcinogens, toxic substances, and respiratory irritants.

62. C: The uniform is not considered PPE. PPE must be supplied without cost to employees and includes gowns and gloves. The face is particularly vulnerable to splashing and splattering of blood and body fluids. Goggles should be non-vented or indirectly vented with an anti-fog coating and solid side shields and should allow for direct and peripheral vision. They should be large enough to cover eyeglasses if necessary and still fit snugly to provide protection. Face shields provide protection to the eyes and face. The shields should have both crown and chin protection and extend around the face to the ears.

63. D: If a female patient's medical history includes "Para 2, gravida 3," this means that the patient has had 2 deliveries of live or stillborn fetus/neonate after 20 weeks gestation and 3 total pregnancies, regardless of duration. Other common terms include:

Nulligravida	A woman who has never been pregnant.
Primigravida	A woman with her first pregnancy.
Multigravida	A woman in her 2nd or later pregnancy.
Nullipara	Woman who has not given birth after 20 weeks gestation
Primipara	A woman who has given birth, live or stillborn, one time at greater than 20 weeks gestation.
Multipara	A woman who has given birth, live or stillborn, equal to or greater than 2 times at greater than 20 weeks gestation.
Grand multipara	A woman who has given birth, live or stillborn, equal to or greater than 5 times at greater than 20 weeks gestation.

64. A: When taking a patient's temperature with an electronic ear (tympanic) thermometer, the temperature usually registers within 2 seconds. It's important to cover the tip with a disposable cover and to point the tip toward the tympanic membrane (eardrum) in order to obtain an accurate reading. Waxy buildup in the ear may interfere with the temperature reading. Ear thermometers are especially useful for small children who cannot hold a thermometer in their mouths and who may resist rectal temperatures.

65. B: Section B is the epigastric region:

A: Right hypochondriac
B: Epigastric (Epi = on, above)
C: Left hypochondriac
D: Right lumbar
E: Umbilical
F: Left lumbar
G: Right iliac
H: Hypogastric (Hypo = below, beneath, less than normal)
I: Left iliac

66. D: If a patient is severely hearing impaired but is able to read lips fairly well and has slight hearing from hearing aids, the CMAA should speak slowly and clearly from three to six feet, facing

the patient, and use gestures to augment communication (but not excessively). The CMAA should avoid speaking loudly and should verify that the patient is understanding the communication. If patient is given instructions, these should also be provided in writing.

67. B: The correct plural for *vertebra* is *vertebrae*. The same plural rule holds true for axilla (axillae) and sclera (sclerae). Other plural rules include:

-um to -a	bacterium, diverticulum	bacteria, diverticula
-us to -i	thrombus, embolus, bronchus	thrombi, emboli, bronchi (Exceptions: corpus/corpora, meatus/meatus, viscus/viscera, plexus, plexuses)
-is to -es	metastasis, testis, diagnosis	metastases, testes, diagnoses (Exceptions: epididymis/epididymides, femur/femora, iris/irides)
-ma or -oma to -mata	carcinoma, fibroma, condyloma	carcinomata, fibromata, condylomata (Note: simply adding -s is now also acceptable)
-ax, -ix, and -yx to -ces	thorax, appendix, calyx	thoraces, appendices, calyces
-nx to -nges	pharynx, phalanx	pharynges, phalanges

68. C: When a new patient checks in, the CMAA should confirm identity with two forms of ID with at least one a photo ID, such as a passport, driver's license, military ID, Native American tribal ID, or federal, state, or local government ID. At subsequent visits, patients are usually asked their name and birthdate although some require photo IDs at each visit or if any information is requested. Some practices now take photos of all patients with their permission and place them in the medical records to further verify ID.

69. A: When scheduling diagnostic procedures for a patient, the CMAA should first verify that services are covered under the patient's insurance plan. If information on the patient's insurance card is not adequate, then the CMAA may need to contact the insurance company by telephone. In some cases, preauthorization may be required for procedures. Once the appointment is made, the patient should be advised of any pre-test and post-test instructions and the procedure noted in the patient's medical record and the diagnostic procedure tracking log.

70. D: The best method of obtaining copayment from a patient is to state: "How would you like to make your $20.00 copayment?" This informs the patient of the amount, the need to pay, and assumes the patient will do so. Copayments are usually collected when the patient checks in although some practices may collect the copayment when the patient checks out. The CMAA should provide a receipt for all cash payments and for check payments on request of the patient. If paying by credit card, the CMAA should make sure that the patient signs the payment receipt and retains a copy.

71. C: If the answering machine shows four patients called requesting visits, the patient with the most acute problem should be scheduled first. In this case W. Barrett has flu and a cough with increasing shortness of breath, which could indicate a complication such as pneumonia. S. Locke, with abdominal pain and cramping, may receive instructions for home care by the physician. Both T. Stanton (urinary frequency and burning) and E. Nehlich (memory loss) should be scheduled with T. Stanton's needs more acute than E. Nehlich's.

72. D: If a patient responds to the CMAA slowly and in very broken English, the CMAA should ask what language the patient speaks at home and if the patient can understand. Patients are often able

to understand more than their speech would indicate. Using simple language and speaking somewhat slowly and clearly may help with the patient's comprehension. Gesture and pictures, if available, may help with communication as well. It's important to remember that patients may be very intelligent but simply lacking in English skills.

73. B: If a patient by the name of Jennifer Brown presents this insurance card at a visit, the most likely reason is that that the patient is covered under Mary Jones' family plan. Cards may vary with some cards listing all covered members. Some may issue separate cards to family members with each card listing the individual's name and/or ID number. In some cases, the CMAA may have to verify coverage with the insurance company.

74. C: If paper health records are filed using terminal digit filing and a patient's health record is numbered 44-62-10, the chart will be filed in section 10 as the last digits are the primary set of numbers referred to for filing purposes, and the middle set (62) is the secondary set, indicating the correct subsection in section 10. The chart will be placed between charts 43 and 45 in subsection 62 in section 10. Other filing methods include straight numeric filing, alphanumeric filing (initials of patient precede number), and middle digit filing.

75. C: If a patient is part of an HMO and needs a regular (non-emergent) referral to see a specialist, gaining approval usually takes 3 to 10 days although this varies according to the carrier. If the physician indicates that the referral is urgent (but non-life threatening, approval is usually received within 24 hours. For stat (emergent) referrals, approval should be received within a few minutes to an hour.

76. D: If, in the waiting area where other patients are present, the CMAA asks a patient the reason for his visit, this is an example of a HIPAA violation. The patient's reason for seeking medical care is a confidential matter and cannot be shared with those who are unauthorized to receive the information. Asking for this information in public puts the patient in an uncomfortable situation. The only information that should be expressed within the hearing of others is the patient's name or unique identifier.

77. D: The purpose of an Advance Beneficiary Notice is to notify patients that a service may not be covered by Medicare. The services in question should be itemized and the reason provided. The estimated cost of the services should also be included in the notice so that a patient can make an informed decision about whether to proceed and pay for the services. Usually the form has two options: "Yes" to proceed with the services and "No" to not proceed. The form must be dated and signed by the patient.

78. B: If a patient's record indicates that the patient has developed folate (vitamin B-12) deficiency anemia because of long-term use of the drug metformin for diabetic treatment, this means that the condition was caused by the drug metformin, so the correct coding would be: D52.1 Drug-induced folate deficiency anemia. The D52 refers to folate deficiency anemia, and the numeral after the decimal point indicates the specific type. Correct coding is essential for reimbursement. If the cause is unknown, then the unspecified code (D52.9) is utilized.

79. C: The *guarantor* of an account is the person who is responsible for paying bills not paid for by insurance. In some cases, this may be the person for whom the account is established, but in other cases, it may be a parent or other individual. If the patient is not the guarantor of his/her account, then the name, address, and contact information (phone number, email address) of the guarantor must be recorded for billing purposes.

80. D: When setting up user accounts, D36&lobx would be classified as a strong password because it is 8 characters in length and is a combination of uppercase letters, lower case letters, numbers, and symbols. The user should avoid names (such as Carolina or of family members, friends, or animals) or phrases (such as Ilovemycat). Dates should be avoided (such as wedding anniversaries and birthdates 12161980 [12-16-1980]) because they are commonly used and easy to guess.

81. A: This information would be found in the physician's orders. While patient records may vary somewhat from one institution to another, the health record typically includes an admission form with demographic information, history and physical exam report, physician's orders, progress notes (physician, nurse, and other healthcare practitioners as indicated), laboratory reports, pathology reports (if appropriate), medication and treatment records, operative report (if indicated), consultant reports, and discharge summary.

82. B: In terms of filing claims, "bundling" refers to including a number of different procedures under one code. This is commonly done, for example, when the same steps are taken each time for a surgical procedure. Bundling saves time when it comes to coding. In some cases, such as when an unusual event occurs during a bundled procedure, unbundling may be done, but if unbundling is done just to increase payments, then it is a fraudulent practice.

83. A: If a patient tells the CMAA that the physician has recommended the patient see a podiatrist (foot specialist) for nail care and asks whom to see, the CMAA should refer to the practice's list of recommended referrals. Whenever possible, the patient should be provided at least two or three choices. If the practice does not maintain a list, then the CMAA should ask the physician for a recommendation but should not give a personal recommendation.

84. D: A **durable power of attorney** allows the designated person to make all legal decisions for a patient, including decisions about health care, even if the patient remains competent. A **living will** provides instructions to medical staff regarding end-of-life care and may include provisions regarding organ donation. An **advance directive** may include a living will, and DNR, and designation of a healthcare proxy. A **healthcare proxy** designates a person to make decisions about healthcare and DNR if the patient becomes incapable of making the decisions.

85. C: According to this account aging report, two accounts are delinquent: Those of R. Moore and M. Shaw because both of those accounts have not been reimbursed for more than 30 days. The account of T. Jones is current and not yet overdue. The **accounts aging record** is used to track insurance payments, including those that are past due. The aging of accounts is done by 30-day increments (0-30, 31-60, etc.). Unless a payment agreement has been agreed upon in advance, all payments are considered past due after 30 days. Those that exceed 120 days are usually referred to a collection agency or written off by the practice.

86. D: In a tickler file, a copy of a submitted claim is generally placed under the day that is 6 weeks after the submission date. If the account has not been reimbursed by that date, it is delinquent and a follow-up letter should be sent to the insurance company and a notation of that made in the insurance claim register and the claim form and copy of the letter advanced an additional 2 to 6 weeks in the tickler file. The contents of the tickler file should be reviewed at the end of each billing period to determine if any submissions have not yet been paid or are overdue.

87. B: A pre-invoice is used to provide an estimate of costs of services. The pre-invoice is often given to the patient before or after procedures are scheduled to alert the patient to any charges for which the patient may be responsible. An invoice, on the other hand, is the billing form that lists

and describes the purchases or services, the fee, any payments received, and the balance due as well as the date at which the payment is due.

88. A: An example of correct ergonomics is to hold weight (such as when carrying a box) close to the body rather than at arm's length. The CMAA should avoid pulling but should push, roll, or slide instead and should flex at the knees and hips rather than the waist when lifting an item. The CMAA should avoid reaching overhead for prolonged periods of time or for more than 20 inches. The CMAA should maintain a firm base of support with feet apart and should not hesitate to get help.

89. D: When screening a patient over the telephone, it is essential that the CMAA follow a screening manual so the questions are consistent with the type of complaint. State regulations regarding screening by unlicensed personnel vary from state to state, but CMAAs are usually allowed to screen calls with training in asking appropriate questions. The screening manual should list the appropriate questions to ask depending on the patient's complaints/issues and indicate which responses require intervention of other healthcare providers, such as an RN or emergency medical personnel (9-1-1).

90. C: If a CMAA receives a needlestick injury from a needle and syringe inadvertently thrown into the trash, the first step should be to thoroughly wash the area with soap and water. Then, the CMAA should report the injury to a supervisor, ensure the injury is entered, as required by law, into the needles and sharps injury log, and seek medical attention. If possible, the patient source should be identified and the need for prophylactic treatment (such as for HIV) determined.

91. B: If a physician bills for a service at a higher level than that actually provided, this is an example of upcoding. This increases reimbursement but is an act of fraud. Downcoding occurs when lower level codes are used for higher level procedures or services. Upcoding is most often carried out by healthcare providers and downcoding by insurance claims examiners. Downcoding may occur when the description of a procedure or service in the medical records does not match the CPT code.

92. A: If a chemical spills in the office, before cleaning up the spill, the CMAA should immediately consult the Safety Data Sheet (SDS) (formerly Material Safety Data Sheet) to learn how to handle the substance and about the toxic effects. SDSs for common chemical and products used in the practice should be readily available as well as any neutralizing substances that may be needed. Manufacturers and suppliers should have SDSs on file and can be contacted for copies. OSHA/EPA Occupational Chemical Database provides links for SDSs for some products.

93. A: If a physician routinely bills for a comprehensive exam for all Medicare patients, regardless of their symptoms or complaints, this is an example of Medicare fraud because the exam is not, in call cases, necessary. The four types of Medicare fraud include:

- Billing for services not actually provided.
- Billing for patients not actually seen.
- Billing for unnecessary services, procedures, and tests.
- Upcoding.

Whistleblowers are protected by law and may be eligible for a reward.

94. C: OSHA's general duty clause states that the workplace may be free of hazards that may result in harm. Because the law does not itemize every possible infraction or hazard, the general duty clause serves as a blanket clause to cover all general possibilities that are not otherwise covered. OSHA requires medical facilities to comply with bloodborne pathogen standards, including

providing personal protective equipment, and to have documented proof of compliance. Emergency evacuation plans must also be in place.

95. D: If the physician has ordered that a patient enter an alcohol rehabilitation program, but the patient refuses to do so, the patient is exercising the right to refuse treatment under the Right to Self-Determination Act. Patients have the right to refuse care, but the refusal must be documented in the patient's medical record. This is especially important if the refusal puts the patient's health at risk. Parents also have the right to refuse care for their minor children.

96. B: When a patient makes an appointment to see a physician and allows the CMAA to take vital signs without expressly giving permission, this is an example of implied consent. Minor procedures, such as vital signs, ear lavage, and phlebotomy are generally covered by implied consent (meaning that the patient would not make the appointment without expecting some procedures be carried out) and can be done without a separate consent form, but major procedures, such as a colonoscopy, require informed consent.

97. C: If a staff member takes $20 from petty cash to buy coffee and tea for the breakroom, the CMAA should log it into the petty cash record and give the staff member a petty cash receipt. The petty cash record should include any disbursements and replenishments. Petty cash should be kept in a locked secure place, such as a drawer. Petty cash usually consists of less than $100 and is used for miscellaneous costs, such as parking costs, postage, tips for delivery persons, and breakroom supplies.

98. A: If a physician refuses to treat a patient with severe disabilities because of the inconvenience caused by needing to use special lifts and equipment, the physician is in violation of the ADA (Americans with Disabilities Act). Additionally, the facility must be accessible with ramps for wheelchairs, accessible door handles, accessible bathrooms and drinking fountains, and elevators (multi-story buildings). An examining room must be available that allows space for a wheelchair.

99. D: If a nurse claims to have forgotten his/her password and asks to use the CMAA's password to access a patient's electronic health record (EHR), the CMAA should refuse to allow the nurse to use the password: 'I'm sorry, but I can't legally allow someone else to use my password." The CMAA should also refuse to access the EHR to allow the nurse to view it because an audit trail would show the CMAA accessed the record and not the nurse.

100. B: Medicaid is a combined federal and state welfare program to assist people with low incomes with payment for medical care. Rules and benefits vary from one state to another. Some states have expanded Medicaid to cover more low-income individuals. This program provides assistance for all ages, including children. Older adults receiving SSI are eligible as are others who meet state eligibility requirements. Also, older adults on Medicare may receive Medicaid as a secondary insurance.

101. C: **CMS-1500** (AKA HCFA-1500) is the medical claim form generally used by physicians and out-patient medical practices as well as various types of therapy practices and out-patient programs. CMS-1500 was developed by Medicare but is now used as a standard by others in the insurance industry. **CMS-1450** (AKA UB-04), on the other hand, is aimed at institutions and utilized by hospitals and other types of inpatient facilities for billing.

102. B: This sign-in sheet is not HIPAA compliant because it contains identifying information: the patient's birthdate. Sign in sheets are covered by the HIPAA Privacy rule and may contain the date and time of arrival, the patient's name, the appointment time, and the health providers name. Any

additional information asked for, such as whether the patient is a new patient, must not include protected health information (PHI).

103. C: Patients should be apprised of all reasonable risks and any complications or adverse effects, such as post-procedure pain, as well as benefits. Providing informed consent is a requirement of all states. Informed consent must be signed by the patient or guardian prior to procedures and should include:

- Explanation of diagnosis.
- Nature and reason for treatment or procedure.
- Risks and benefits.
- Alternative options (regardless of cost or insurance coverage).
- Risks and benefits of alternative options.
- Risks and benefits of not having a treatment or procedure.

104. A: The out-of-pocket amount that Medicare recipients are required to pay each year before Medicare starts paying is the *deductible*. There is a deductible for both parts A and B and it changes from year to year. For example, in 2019, Medicare A deductible is $1364 and Medicare B deductible is $185 although secondary insurance may, in fact, pay some of these charges. Many other insurance policies also require a deductible, and the deductible may be in the thousands of dollars for less costly insurance policies.

105. C: The dollar amount that an insurance company considers payment in full for a claim is the *allowed amount*. For example, an insurance company may pay only $300 for an MRI that costs $800. If the insurance company has negotiated a discount, the balance may be written off by the provider. However, if not, the insured may be responsible for the balance of a claim, or a secondary insurance may cover all or part of the balance.

106. B: If a CMAA must create a number of different documents (letters, calendar, fax cover sheet) in a word processing program, the first step should be to search for templates. A template is a preformatted file that is document-ready so that margins and headings and basic format do not need to be created but only the text added. Word processing programs, such as MS Word offer a number of different templates, and thousands are available online, many of them without cost. Using a template can save considerable time.

107. A: If first-class postage for an envelope weighing up to one ounce is $0.55, then an envelope weighing 1.5 ounces requires postage of $0.70 because each additional ounce after the first costs $0.15. Postcards cost $0.35. Many practices used metered stamps, which print on the envelope, because they send out large volumes of mail, and metering is more efficient than applying individual stamps. Additionally, the cost of metered mail for letters is discounted to $0.50 with $0.15 for each additional ounce.

108. A: If a medical practice uses electronic health records and has an image-based backup system for both local and distant backup, the backups should ideally be done every hour to limit the amount of data that may be lost if, for example, the computer system goes down. Image-based systems essentially take a picture of all programs and files so that they can easily be restored. This is especially important if a virus infects a program or system or files become corrupted.

109. C: If a CMAA is faxing sensitive information about a patient to another healthcare provider, the most important action is for the CMAA to call ahead to say the fax is coming and to ensure an appropriate person is there to receive the fax so it doesn't stay at the machine. The CMAA should

- 144 -

also verify receipt of the fax and mark it is as "confidential." Records sent from one healthcare provider to another and covered by a medical release do not need to be deidentified.

110. B: If a CMAA sees that another staff member has posted a picture of a patient on Facebook with negative comments about the patient's weight and mental health issues, the CMAA should immediately report it to a supervisor at the practice as this is not only a HIPAA violation but also an ethical violation. The CMAA should not discuss it with the staff member or attempt to intervene. Even if the entry is taken down, someone may have a copy. It is the responsibility of the practice to report the matter and deal with the staff person.

111. D: While ideally someone should always be at a front desk to welcome and check-in patients, in small practices, this is not always possible. In this case, the best solution is likely to post a sign asking patients to sign in and take a seat because some patients may be confused about what to do (leave or stay) if no one is at the desk. Playing an audio greeting repeatedly may become very annoying to those waiting.

112. B: The purpose of a firewall (a network security device) is to block unauthorized access to computer programs. The firewall prevents external sources, such as a website on the Internet, from entering the network system and corrupting data. A firewall may comprise software, hardware, or both. All medical practices should have firewalls in place to protect their computer systems and prevent unauthorized access to patient's electronic medical records.

113. B: If a new patient is scheduled two weeks in the future, the CMAA should mail the demographic form to the patient to fill out before the visit. Some practices also post a downloadable document on line, but return is usually better if the documents are mailed rather than expecting the patient to find the document, download, and print it, and not all patients have access to a computer or know how to carry out common functions.

114. C: If the CMAA is typing a letter in MS Word and accidentally deletes a paragraph, the CMAA should select the "undo typing" command or button (backward facing curved arrow) which will undo the last actions. MS Word automatically saves the last 100 actions. However, if the user carries out a save after an action, the action cannot be retrieved with the undo command. Thus, if the CMAA accidentally deleted the file and then selected "save," the deleted portion is lost.

115. B: The primary advantage of just-in-time ordering of inventory is cost saving. Ordering is done only when the supply of an item is almost depleted, so less money is tied up in inventory on hand. Additionally, there is less chance that supplies will become outdated so there is less loss. Ordering may also be done automatically when a stock item reaches a certain level, especially when inventory is computerized, saving both time and labor.

116. D: Gross negligence. Type of negligence include:

- Negligent conduct: Failure to provide reasonable care or to protect/assist another, based on standards and expertise.
- Gross negligence: Willful provision of inadequate care with disregard for the safety and security of another.
- Contributory negligence: Injured party contributes to his/her own harm.
- Comparative negligence: Attributes percentage amount of negligence to each individual involved.

117. A: If a patient with a history of mental disease begins swearing and pacing back and forth in the waiting area, yelling, "You can't make me stay here!" the best initial response is to speak calmly

and quietly to the patient. The CMAA should remain in control and avoid reactions that suggest fear or anger. The CMAA should stand if sitting but avoid moving aggressively toward the patient but should move away if the situation appears to be escalating and it is safe to do so and other patients are not in the area.

118. D: When entering the examining room of a patient who is deaf and facing away from the door, the CMAA should clap or tap the foot. Patients who are deaf are often more sensitive to vibrations, so this will likely alert them that someone is present. If there is no response, the CMAA should try to approach from the direction the patient is facing in order to avoid startling the patient by touching the patient from behind.

119. C: When the physician is almost ready to see a patient, the CMAA should generally place the patient's medical record in the file holder with the name facing inward although it is not a HIPAA violation to have the name exposed. Keeping the name facing inward prevents other patients traversing the hall from knowing which patient is in that examining room. Records should not be left in the patient's examining room as the patient or family members may read through them or take pages.

120. B: When using a computer, the monitor should be adjusted so that the user's eyes are in a line that is 2 to 3 inches below the top of the monitor casing with viewing distance of approximately the length of the user's arm as this distance generally allows the user to view the entire monitor without moving the head from side to side, which can cause muscle strain. The arms should be bent to about 90 degrees at the elbows with the hands and wrist in straight alignment.

121. D: A nonverbal clue that a client may be anxious is if the client rubs the hands together constantly as this is a self-comforting measure. Nonverbal behavior can include the tone of voice and cadence of speech, body positioning or behaviors (arms crossed, sitting forward, leaning backward), facial expressions (frowning, grimacing, relaxed), eye cast, amount of eye contact, obvious autonomic physiological responses (diaphoresis and blushing), personal appearance (grooming, hygiene), and physical characteristics (extreme over- or under-weight).

122. A: "The law doesn't allow me to give out any information about patients in order to protect their privacy and safety" is accurate and appropriate. The Health Insurance Portability and Accountability Act (HIPAA) addresses the privacy of health information. The CMAA must not release any information or documentation about a patient's condition or treatment without consent. Failure to comply with HIPAA regulations can make a CMAA liable for legal action.

123. C: In MS Excel, the best function for adding up all of the values in a column is SUM. Excel is a software spreadsheet application that organizes and stores data (numeric or text) in tables and allows for analysis. Cells in a spreadsheet are arranged in columns and rows. Spreadsheets were originally used primarily for budgetary reasons to track income and expenditures, but use has expanded. For example, Excel may be utilized to keep records of inventory.

124. D: If the CMAA is using the PASS acronym to guide use of a fire extinguisher, the letters stand for:

P = **P**ull the pin of the fire extinguisher.
A = **A**im the nozzle at the fire.
S = **S**queeze the handle of the fire extinguisher.
S = **S**pray from side to side, starting at the base of the fire.

For any fire, the fire department should be called per 9-1-1, and staff members should not attempt to put out a fire that is large or dangerous although they may use the extinguisher against a small fire, such as in a wastebasket. The primary concern must always be the safety of the patients and staff.

125. A: When closing the office at the end of the day, the first task should be to make sure that all staff, visitors, and patients have gone by checking in all of the rooms, including bathrooms and storage rooms. If a patient has been forgotten and remains behind, the CMAA should escort the patient outside. If the CMAA suspects that an unauthorized person is hiding somewhere in the office or building, the CMAA should immediately call security or the police.

126. C: When writing a letter on paper with a letterhead, the date is generally placed on the third line below the letterhead. If there is no letterhead on the paper, then the date is usually placed at line 13. Business letters always be written on letterhead as it gives a more professional appearance. Margins are generally one inch on the right and left sides although they may be wider if the letter is very short.

127. D: The CMAA should sent the letter by certified mail:

Mail options: USPS	
First class	Mail delivery for items weighing 12 ounces or less.
Certified	Sender receives a receipt and receiver must sign to receive mail/package. Tracking available. Proof of delivery maintained for 2 years by USPS. Return Receipt (proof of delivery) can be purchased. May take up to 5 days for delivery.
Registered	Similar to certified but transported per locked or sealed containers and tracking available. Insurance can be purchased for up to $25,000. May take up to 15 days for delivery.
Priority	Mail delivery for items weighing 13 ounces to 70 pounds.

128. A: Purging of files refers to moving a file from active to inactive. Patient files are generally classified as active (those patients still being seen), inactive (patients who have not seen the physician for 6 months to a year or longer), and closed (patients who have terminated care, moved out of the area, or are deceased). If stickers are placed on the files indicating the last year the patient visited the physician, then purging, which should be done at least annually, can be carried out easily by simply checking the date stickers.

129. A: Current Procedural Terminology (CPT) was developed by the American Medical Association (AMA) and is used to code for medical procedures and services under health insurance plans (both public and private). The code set is copyrighted by the AMA and is continually evaluated and updated annually in October of each year. Medicare utilizes an adjusted form of CPT, the HCPS code. While ICD-10 codes are used to code for procedures, ICD-10 coding is used only for inpatients.

HHS has designed CPT codes as part of the national standard for electronic healthcare transactions:

- Category I: Identify a procedure or service.
- Category II: Identify performance measures, including diagnostic procedures.
- Category III: Identify temporary codes for technology and data collection.

130. D: The correct alphabetical order is:

- Trudy Santa Maria
- S.C. Smith (initials go before names starting with the same letter).
- Sam C. Smith.
- Jacob Smithson. (short forms, such as Smith, go before long)
- Dana Synder
- Sara St. John (commonly used abbreviated forms, such as St. are used as written).

How to Overcome Test Anxiety

Just the thought of taking a test is enough to make most people a little nervous. A test is an important event that can have a long-term impact on your future, so it's important to take it seriously and it's natural to feel anxious about performing well. But just because anxiety is normal, that doesn't mean that it's helpful in test taking, or that you should simply accept it as part of your life. Anxiety can have a variety of effects. These effects can be mild, like making you feel slightly nervous, or severe, like blocking your ability to focus or remember even a simple detail.

If you experience test anxiety—whether severe or mild—it's important to know how to beat it. To discover this, first you need to understand what causes test anxiety.

Causes of Test Anxiety

While we often think of anxiety as an uncontrollable emotional state, it can actually be caused by simple, practical things. One of the most common causes of test anxiety is that a person does not feel adequately prepared for their test. This feeling can be the result of many different issues such as poor study habits or lack of organization, but the most common culprit is time management. Starting to study too late, failing to organize your study time to cover all of the material, or being distracted while you study will mean that you're not well prepared for the test. This may lead to cramming the night before, which will cause you to be physically and mentally exhausted for the test. Poor time management also contributes to feelings of stress, fear, and hopelessness as you realize you are not well prepared but don't know what to do about it.

Other times, test anxiety is not related to your preparation for the test but comes from unresolved fear. This may be a past failure on a test, or poor performance on tests in general. It may come from comparing yourself to others who seem to be performing better or from the stress of living up to expectations. Anxiety may be driven by fears of the future—how failure on this test would affect your educational and career goals. These fears are often completely irrational, but they can still negatively impact your test performance.

> **Review Video:** 3 Reasons You Have Test Anxiety
> Visit mometrix.com/academy and enter code: 428468

Elements of Test Anxiety

As mentioned earlier, test anxiety is considered to be an emotional state, but it has physical and mental components as well. Sometimes you may not even realize that you are suffering from test anxiety until you notice the physical symptoms. These can include trembling hands, rapid heartbeat, sweating, nausea, and tense muscles. Extreme anxiety may lead to fainting or vomiting. Obviously, any of these symptoms can have a negative impact on testing. It is important to recognize them as soon as they begin to occur so that you can address the problem before it damages your performance.

> **Review Video:** 3 Ways to Tell You Have Test Anxiety
> Visit mometrix.com/academy and enter code: 927847

The mental components of test anxiety include trouble focusing and inability to remember learned information. During a test, your mind is on high alert, which can help you recall information and stay focused for an extended period of time. However, anxiety interferes with your mind's natural processes, causing you to blank out, even on the questions you know well. The strain of testing during anxiety makes it difficult to stay focused, especially on a test that may take several hours. Extreme anxiety can take a huge mental toll, making it difficult not only to recall test information but even to understand the test questions or pull your thoughts together.

> **Review Video:** How Test Anxiety Affects Memory
> Visit mometrix.com/academy and enter code: 609003

Effects of Test Anxiety

Test anxiety is like a disease—if left untreated, it will get progressively worse. Anxiety leads to poor performance, and this reinforces the feelings of fear and failure, which in turn lead to poor performances on subsequent tests. It can grow from a mild nervousness to a crippling condition. If allowed to progress, test anxiety can have a big impact on your schooling, and consequently on your future.

Test anxiety can spread to other parts of your life. Anxiety on tests can become anxiety in any stressful situation, and blanking on a test can turn into panicking in a job situation. But fortunately, you don't have to let anxiety rule your testing and determine your grades. There are a number of relatively simple steps you can take to move past anxiety and function normally on a test and in the rest of life.

> **Review Video:** How Test Anxiety Impacts Your Grades
> Visit mometrix.com/academy and enter code: 939819

Physical Steps for Beating Test Anxiety

While test anxiety is a serious problem, the good news is that it can be overcome. It doesn't have to control your ability to think and remember information. While it may take time, you can begin taking steps today to beat anxiety.

Just as your first hint that you may be struggling with anxiety comes from the physical symptoms, the first step to treating it is also physical. Rest is crucial for having a clear, strong mind. If you are tired, it is much easier to give in to anxiety. But if you establish good sleep habits, your body and mind will be ready to perform optimally, without the strain of exhaustion. Additionally, sleeping well helps you to retain information better, so you're more likely to recall the answers when you see the test questions.

Getting good sleep means more than going to bed on time. It's important to allow your brain time to relax. Take study breaks from time to time so it doesn't get overworked, and don't study right before bed. Take time to rest your mind before trying to rest your body, or you may find it difficult to fall asleep.

> **Review Video: The Importance of Sleep for Your Brain**
> Visit mometrix.com/academy and enter code: 319338

Along with sleep, other aspects of physical health are important in preparing for a test. Good nutrition is vital for good brain function. Sugary foods and drinks may give a burst of energy but this burst is followed by a crash, both physically and emotionally. Instead, fuel your body with protein and vitamin-rich foods.

Also, drink plenty of water. Dehydration can lead to headaches and exhaustion, especially if your brain is already under stress from the rigors of the test. Particularly if your test is a long one, drink water during the breaks. And if possible, take an energy-boosting snack to eat between sections.

> **Review Video: How Diet Can Affect your Mood**
> Visit mometrix.com/academy and enter code: 624317

Along with sleep and diet, a third important part of physical health is exercise. Maintaining a steady workout schedule is helpful, but even taking 5-minute study breaks to walk can help get your blood pumping faster and clear your head. Exercise also releases endorphins, which contribute to a positive feeling and can help combat test anxiety.

When you nurture your physical health, you are also contributing to your mental health. If your body is healthy, your mind is much more likely to be healthy as well. So take time to rest, nourish your body with healthy food and water, and get moving as much as possible. Taking these physical steps will make you stronger and more able to take the mental steps necessary to overcome test anxiety.

> **Review Video: How to Stay Healthy and Prevent Test Anxiety**
> Visit mometrix.com/academy and enter code: 877894

Mental Steps for Beating Test Anxiety

Working on the mental side of test anxiety can be more challenging, but as with the physical side, there are clear steps you can take to overcome it. As mentioned earlier, test anxiety often stems from lack of preparation, so the obvious solution is to prepare for the test. Effective studying may be the most important weapon you have for beating test anxiety, but you can and should employ several other mental tools to combat fear.

First, boost your confidence by reminding yourself of past success—tests or projects that you aced. If you're putting as much effort into preparing for this test as you did for those, there's no reason you should expect to fail here. Work hard to prepare; then trust your preparation.

Second, surround yourself with encouraging people. It can be helpful to find a study group, but be sure that the people you're around will encourage a positive attitude. If you spend time with others who are anxious or cynical, this will only contribute to your own anxiety. Look for others who are motivated to study hard from a desire to succeed, not from a fear of failure.

Third, reward yourself. A test is physically and mentally tiring, even without anxiety, and it can be helpful to have something to look forward to. Plan an activity following the test, regardless of the outcome, such as going to a movie or getting ice cream.

When you are taking the test, if you find yourself beginning to feel anxious, remind yourself that you know the material. Visualize successfully completing the test. Then take a few deep, relaxing breaths and return to it. Work through the questions carefully but with confidence, knowing that you are capable of succeeding.

Developing a healthy mental approach to test taking will also aid in other areas of life. Test anxiety affects more than just the actual test—it can be damaging to your mental health and even contribute to depression. It's important to beat test anxiety before it becomes a problem for more than testing.

> **Review Video: Test Anxiety and Depression**
> Visit mometrix.com/academy and enter code: 904704

Study Strategy

Being prepared for the test is necessary to combat anxiety, but what does being prepared look like? You may study for hours on end and still not feel prepared. What you need is a strategy for test prep. The next few pages outline our recommended steps to help you plan out and conquer the challenge of preparation.

Step 1: Scope Out the Test

Learn everything you can about the format (multiple choice, essay, etc.) and what will be on the test. Gather any study materials, course outlines, or sample exams that may be available. Not only will this help you to prepare, but knowing what to expect can help to alleviate test anxiety.

Step 2: Map Out the Material

Look through the textbook or study guide and make note of how many chapters or sections it has. Then divide these over the time you have. For example, if a book has 15 chapters and you have five days to study, you need to cover three chapters each day. Even better, if you have the time, leave an extra day at the end for overall review after you have gone through the material in depth.

If time is limited, you may need to prioritize the material. Look through it and make note of which sections you think you already have a good grasp on, and which need review. While you are studying, skim quickly through the familiar sections and take more time on the challenging parts. Write out your plan so you don't get lost as you go. Having a written plan also helps you feel more in control of the study, so anxiety is less likely to arise from feeling overwhelmed at the amount to cover.

Step 3: Gather Your Tools

Decide what study method works best for you. Do you prefer to highlight in the book as you study and then go back over the highlighted portions? Or do you type out notes of the important information? Or is it helpful to make flashcards that you can carry with you? Assemble the pens, index cards, highlighters, post-it notes, and any other materials you may need so you won't be distracted by getting up to find things while you study.

If you're having a hard time retaining the information or organizing your notes, experiment with different methods. For example, try color-coding by subject with colored pens, highlighters, or post-it notes. If you learn better by hearing, try recording yourself reading your notes so you can listen while in the car, working out, or simply sitting at your desk. Ask a friend to quiz you from your flashcards, or try teaching someone the material to solidify it in your mind.

Step 4: Create Your Environment

It's important to avoid distractions while you study. This includes both the obvious distractions like visitors and the subtle distractions like an uncomfortable chair (or a too-comfortable couch that makes you want to fall asleep). Set up the best study environment possible: good lighting and a comfortable work area. If background music helps you focus, you may want to turn it on, but otherwise keep the room quiet. If you are using a computer to take notes, be sure you don't have any other windows open, especially applications like social media, games, or anything else that could distract you. Silence your phone and turn off notifications. Be sure to keep water close by so you stay hydrated while you study (but avoid unhealthy drinks and snacks).

Also, take into account the best time of day to study. Are you freshest first thing in the morning? Try to set aside some time then to work through the material. Is your mind clearer in the afternoon or evening? Schedule your study session then. Another method is to study at the same time of day that you will take the test, so that your brain gets used to working on the material at that time and will be ready to focus at test time.

Step 5: Study!

Once you have done all the study preparation, it's time to settle into the actual studying. Sit down, take a few moments to settle your mind so you can focus, and begin to follow your study plan. Don't give in to distractions or let yourself procrastinate. This is your time to prepare so you'll be ready to fearlessly approach the test. Make the most of the time and stay focused.

Of course, you don't want to burn out. If you study too long you may find that you're not retaining the information very well. Take regular study breaks. For example, taking five minutes out of every hour to walk briskly, breathing deeply and swinging your arms, can help your mind stay fresh.

As you get to the end of each chapter or section, it's a good idea to do a quick review. Remind yourself of what you learned and work on any difficult parts. When you feel that you've mastered the material, move on to the next part. At the end of your study session, briefly skim through your notes again.

But while review is helpful, cramming last minute is NOT. If at all possible, work ahead so that you won't need to fit all your study into the last day. Cramming overloads your brain with more information than it can process and retain, and your tired mind may struggle to recall even previously learned information when it is overwhelmed with last-minute study. Also, the urgent nature of cramming and the stress placed on your brain contribute to anxiety. You'll be more likely to go to the test feeling unprepared and having trouble thinking clearly.

So don't cram, and don't stay up late before the test, even just to review your notes at a leisurely pace. Your brain needs rest more than it needs to go over the information again. In fact, plan to finish your studies by noon or early afternoon the day before the test. Give your brain the rest of the day to relax or focus on other things, and get a good night's sleep. Then you will be fresh for the test and better able to recall what you've studied.

Step 6: Take a practice test

Many courses offer sample tests, either online or in the study materials. This is an excellent resource to check whether you have mastered the material, as well as to prepare for the test format and environment.

Check the test format ahead of time: the number of questions, the type (multiple choice, free response, etc.), and the time limit. Then create a plan for working through them. For example, if you have 30 minutes to take a 60-question test, your limit is 30 seconds per question. Spend less time on the questions you know well so that you can take more time on the difficult ones.

If you have time to take several practice tests, take the first one open book, with no time limit. Work through the questions at your own pace and make sure you fully understand them. Gradually work up to taking a test under test conditions: sit at a desk with all study materials put away and set a timer. Pace yourself to make sure you finish the test with time to spare and go back to check your answers if you have time.

After each test, check your answers. On the questions you missed, be sure you understand why you missed them. Did you misread the question (tests can use tricky wording)? Did you forget the information? Or was it something you hadn't learned? Go back and study any shaky areas that the practice tests reveal.

Taking these tests not only helps with your grade, but also aids in combating test anxiety. If you're already used to the test conditions, you're less likely to worry about it, and working through tests until you're scoring well gives you a confidence boost. Go through the practice tests until you feel comfortable, and then you can go into the test knowing that you're ready for it.

Test Tips

On test day, you should be confident, knowing that you've prepared well and are ready to answer the questions. But aside from preparation, there are several test day strategies you can employ to maximize your performance.

First, as stated before, get a good night's sleep the night before the test (and for several nights before that, if possible). Go into the test with a fresh, alert mind rather than staying up late to study.

Try not to change too much about your normal routine on the day of the test. It's important to eat a nutritious breakfast, but if you normally don't eat breakfast at all, consider eating just a protein bar. If you're a coffee drinker, go ahead and have your normal coffee. Just make sure you time it so that the caffeine doesn't wear off right in the middle of your test. Avoid sugary beverages, and drink enough water to stay hydrated but not so much that you need a restroom break 10 minutes into the test. If your test isn't first thing in the morning, consider going for a walk or doing a light workout before the test to get your blood flowing.

Allow yourself enough time to get ready, and leave for the test with plenty of time to spare so you won't have the anxiety of scrambling to arrive in time. Another reason to be early is to select a good seat. It's helpful to sit away from doors and windows, which can be distracting. Find a good seat, get out your supplies, and settle your mind before the test begins.

When the test begins, start by going over the instructions carefully, even if you already know what to expect. Make sure you avoid any careless mistakes by following the directions.

Then begin working through the questions, pacing yourself as you've practiced. If you're not sure on an answer, don't spend too much time on it, and don't let it shake your confidence. Either skip it and come back later, or eliminate as many wrong answers as possible and guess among the remaining ones. Don't dwell on these questions as you continue—put them out of your mind and focus on what lies ahead.

Be sure to read all of the answer choices, even if you're sure the first one is the right answer. Sometimes you'll find a better one if you keep reading. But don't second-guess yourself if you do immediately know the answer. Your gut instinct is usually right. Don't let test anxiety rob you of the information you know.

If you have time at the end of the test (and if the test format allows), go back and review your answers. Be cautious about changing any, since your first instinct tends to be correct, but make sure you didn't misread any of the questions or accidentally mark the wrong answer choice. Look over any you skipped and make an educated guess.

At the end, leave the test feeling confident. You've done your best, so don't waste time worrying about your performance or wishing you could change anything. Instead, celebrate the successful completion of this test. And finally, use this test to learn how to deal with anxiety even better next time.

Review Video: 5 Tips to Beat Test Anxiety
Visit mometrix.com/academy and enter code: 570656

Important Qualification

Not all anxiety is created equal. If your test anxiety is causing major issues in your life beyond the classroom or testing center, or if you are experiencing troubling physical symptoms related to your anxiety, it may be a sign of a serious physiological or psychological condition. If this sounds like your situation, we strongly encourage you to seek professional help.

Thank You

We at Mometrix would like to extend our heartfelt thanks to you, our friend and patron, for allowing us to play a part in your journey. It is a privilege to serve people from all walks of life who are unified in their commitment to building the best future they can for themselves.

The preparation you devote to these important testing milestones may be the most valuable educational opportunity you have for making a real difference in your life. We encourage you to put your heart into it—that feeling of succeeding, overcoming, and yes, conquering will be well worth the hours you've invested.

We want to hear your story, your struggles and your successes, and if you see any opportunities for us to improve our materials so we can help others even more effectively in the future, please share that with us as well. **The team at Mometrix would be absolutely thrilled to hear from you!** So please, send us an email (support@mometrix.com) and let's stay in touch.

If you'd like some additional help, check out these other resources we offer for your exam:

http://MometrixFlashcards.com/cmaa

Additional Bonus Material

Due to our efforts to try to keep this book to a manageable length, we've created a link that will give you access to all of your additional bonus material.

Please visit https://www.mometrix.com/bonus948/cmaa to access the information.